THE MYOCARDIAL CELL

FOR THE

CLINICAL CARDIOLOGIST

by

Marianne J. Legato, M.D.

Assistant Professor of Medicine, Columbia University
College of Physicians and Surgeons

Attending Physician, Department of Medicine,
Roosevelt Hospital, New York

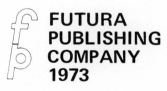
FUTURA
PUBLISHING
COMPANY
1973

Copyright © 1973 by Futura Publishing Company, Inc.

Published by
Futura Publishing Company, Inc.
295 Main Street
Mount Kisco, New York 10549

LC: 73-80701
ISBN: 0-87993-024-1

Printed in U.S.A. by
NOBLE OFFSET PRINTERS, INC.
New York, N.Y. 10003

For

M. Irené Ferrer, M.D.

"Date ei de fructu manuum suarum."
Prov. 31:31.

Acknowledgments

I wish to thank the following people who made invaluable contributions to this book:

Mr. James Burch made with meticulous care the sketches that illustrate the text.

Ms. Roni Fox expertly prepared the material which appears in the electron micrographs.

Ms. Gloria McCord, chief technician in my laboratory, provided technical skills of the highest caliber and in many useful discussions helped to evaluate some of the ideas presented here.

Ms. Felicia Suarez was constantly helpful in general laboratory tasks during the preparation of the manuscript.

Mrs. Gerda Kresse cared for my children with an expertise that fostered an atmosphere essential for the writing of this book.

This work was supported by a grant from the New York Heart Association.

The author is the recipient of a Research Career Development Award from the National Institutes of Health.

Preface

This timely book is a comprehensive, factual, and concise primer of the myocardial cell for the clinical cardiologist. It provides a thorough review and critical appraisal of reported research as well as a lucid exposition of the new advances and persistent problems in myocardial cytology. Stress is placed on information regarding functional and pharmacologic implications of the myocardial cell.

The book, organized under seven main headings, deals effectively with the general anatomy of the myocardial cell, the sarcolemma, and its derivatives, the sarcomere and contractile event, mitochondrion, sarcoplasmic reticulum and relaxation, and myocardial growth and hypertrophy. It concludes with a perspicuous presentation of the atrial, Purkinje, and ventricular cells.

Each chapter incorporates considerable detail into a brief text and is a model of conciseness and economy. The illustrative material, not available in any other book, is of excellent quality and the tables are extremely well planned. Each section concludes with a bibliographic listing of literature which could lead the serious student to original source material for further research.

This book will help physicians bridge the gap between laboratory advances in myocardial cytology and clinical cardiologic practice, and belongs in the library of every cardiologist. It will be an important addition to every reference library.

With this book, Dr. Marianne J. Legato, who has made significant contributions to the knowledge of ultrastructure of the myocardial cell, makes another important contribution to cardiology.

Ephraim Donoso, M.D.

Foreword

This book is a brief summary of the fundamental facts about how the cardiac cell is constructed and how it works in the normal situation. It is intended for the clinical cardiologist. The book was prompted by the fact that research at the level of the myofiber is finding its way with increasing frequency into the literature of clinical cardiology; journals are publishing a substantial number of electron micrographic and electrophysiologic studies which require a knowledge of the normal anatomy of the myofiber and an understanding of what we know and do not know about the role of subcellular systems in the heart. Such work often demands a rather sophisticated level of knowledge for critical appraisal. Hopefully, this monograph will prove useful to the clinician who wishes to evaluate for himself the significance and merit of research at the cellular level.

Marianne J. Legato, M.D.

Table of Contents

CHAPTER I

General Anatomy of the Myocardial Cell

Mammalian myocardium has several characteristics which distinguish it from other types of muscle. It is self-pacing. Its individual fibers contract in a summated or graded rather than an all-or-none fashion. Under normal circumstances it beats synchronously with an almost simultaneous depolarization of all its components in a predictable and orderly fashion.

These special properties of the myocardium are the result of the coordinated activity of a population of muscle cells which is by no means homogeneous. The ordinary working cells of the atria and ventricles, although they all function primarily to develop force in response to an exciting impulse, differ anatomically and electrophysiologically in many important respects. There are specialized cells, whose primary rôles are impulse generation and conduction and not the performance of contractile work; these are the cells unique to the sinus and atrioventricular nodes and the Purkinje cells, with their interesting property of intrinsic rhythmicity and very rapid speed of conduction. It should be emphasized that there are no sharp boundaries between these cell types either anatomically or physiologically: there are transitional cells at the junction between ordinary working myocardial cells and specialized pacing or conducting tissue with anatomic and functional characteristics of both groups. In general, however, there are cells which are structured primarily for the generation or propagation of exciting impulses in the myocardium and cells which are designed principally for the production of contractile force.

In spite of the variations in cardiac cell architecture, there are in all myofibers, as in all muscle cells, three essential physiologic events; excitation, contraction and relaxation. Each of these is produced by the activity of a distinct subcellular system in the myofiber. There is, therefore, a fundamental anatomy common to all the cells of the myocardium, no matter what their rôle in the total economy of the heart.

The myocardial cell, or myofiber, varies in shape from a simple ellipse to a branching cylinder which is many times longer than it is wide (Figure 1 a+b). Its connection with neighboring cells may be sparse and simple, or the cell can be locked into close apposition with the next myofiber by means of an extensive and intricate link peculiar to cardiac tissue known as the *intercalated disc*. Whatever the type of intercellular connection, a significant proportion are electrically low resistance junctions which allow for rapid transmission of impulses from cell to cell, insuring an orderly and virtually simultaneous contraction of all units.

The myofiber has two major tasks: first, it must perform contractile work and second, it must maintain itself. All of the subcellular systems in the myofiber work toward one of these two ends.

Figure 1a. *This is a sketch of a cylindrical, branching cardiac cell or myofiber. It does not represent any particular type of cell, but is meant to show the principal components of the myofiber and their relationship to one another.*

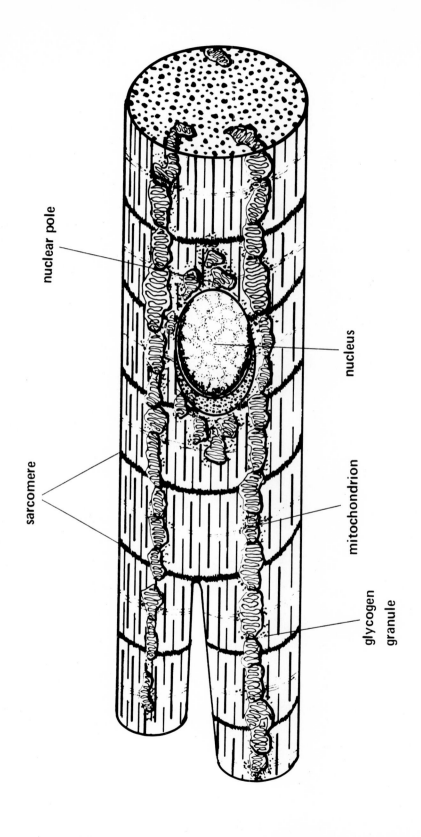

nuclear pole

nucleus

sarcomere

mitochondrion

glycogen
granule

The Myofiber: An Overview

Figure 1b. *This is an electron micrograph of a small section of a ventricular working cell. The section was made parallel to the long axis of the cell. It shows a nucleus (N), the nuclear pole (NP), sarcomeres (S), mitochondria (M), and triadic and diadic units (T, D). L = lipofuscin body. ECS = extracellular space (x 13,300).*

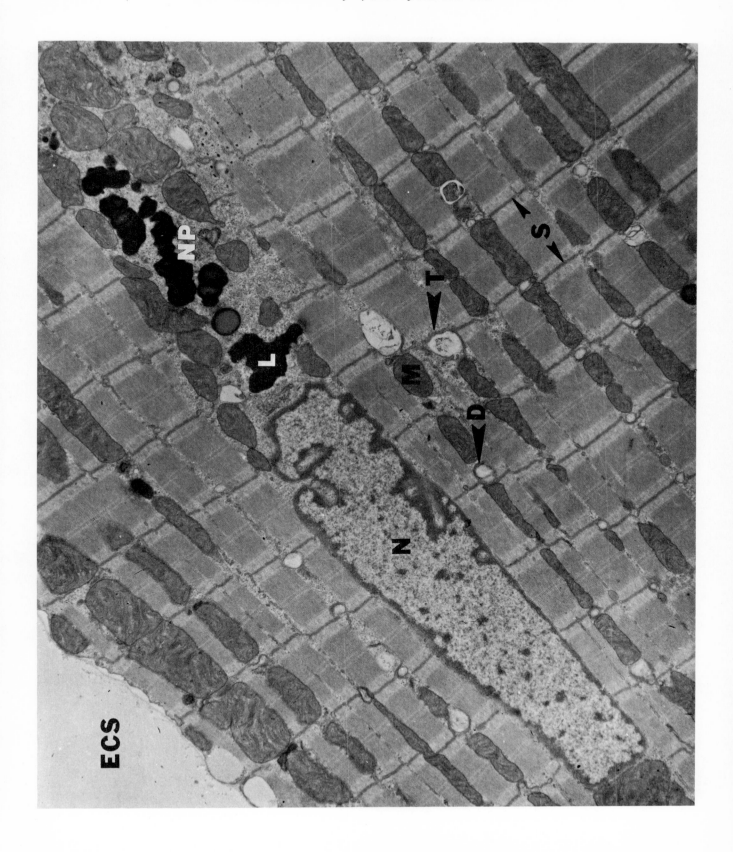

Excitation: The Cell Membrane and its Derivatives

The process of excitation is supported in the cardiac cell, as in all cells, by the cell membrane or *sarcolemma*. In some cells, principally the ordinary working ventricular cell, the sarcolemma is not limited to the surface of the myofiber, but sends invaginating fingers downward and throughout the substance of the sarcoplasm in a system of tubules oriented for the most part perpendicularly to the long axis of the cell (Figure 2). This system of tubules is known collectively as the *transverse tubular system (T-system)* and, by virtue of its continuity with the sarcolemma, expands the area of the surface membrane and carries it downward from the exterior of the cell to all levels of the myofiber. Similarly, in cells with a T-system, the extracellular space is not confined to the cell surface, but extends via the transverse tubular lumen throughout the whole myofiber.

Contraction: The Sarcomere

The bulk of the cell is made up of the contractile units, or *sarcomeres* (Figures 1, 2). These are arranged in long rows called myofibrils which run the entire length of the cell. The sarcomeres are delimited at either end by the electron-dense Z bands into which insert the so-called thin filaments. The latter pass centrally from the Z bands at either side of the sarcomere to interdigitate with a system of thicker filaments occupying the middle of the contractile unit. The resulting pattern of alternating dark and light bands in striated muscle, whether skeletal or cardiac, is the consequence of the arrangement of myofilaments in the sarcomere.

In the resting state, the thin and thick filaments do not interact. When calcium ion is added to the system, cross bridges on the thick filaments make contact with active sites on the thin filaments. It is the sequential making and breaking of these contacts that propels the thin filaments centrally from either end of the sarcomere along the stationary thick filaments, and the Z to Z distance decreases. Calcium ion, then, is the key to the initiation of the contractile event.

Relaxation: The Sarcoplasmic Reticulum

Enveloping the myofibril and thus in intimate contact with the sarcomeres, is a sleeve of intricately branching tubules called the *sarcoplasmic reticulum* (Figure 2). At frequent areas along the sarcolemma and its derivatives, the transverse tubular system and the intercalated disc, the sarcoplasmic tubules flatten out in a specialized cuff of tissue called the lateral sac. The arrangement with regard to the transverse tubular system is such that in many instances the sarcoplasmic reticular network of adjacent sarcomeres each contributes a lateral sac to a transverse tubule; the resulting arrangement, with two lateral sacs parenthesizing a central transverse tubule, is called a triad. If only one lateral sac is present, the configuration is called a diad.

The tubules of the sarcoplasmic reticulum have a well-demonstrated ability to actively pump calcium out of the surrounding environment against a concentration gradient. During the contractile event, when the calcium concentration in the area of the myofilaments reaches a critical level (10^{-7} M) the sarcotubules begin to remove the cation from the area of the sarcomere and return it to an inactive site in the cell, presumably the calcium storage depots of the lateral sac. Interaction between thin and thick filaments stops and the contractile event is over. Relaxation, then, is the function of the sarcotubular network.

The activity of these subcellular systems, which are present in all myofibers, produces the characteristic physiology of the cardiac muscle cell: excitation, achieved as a consequence of sarcolemmal depolarization, releases calcium ion from a superficial site in the cell to the myofilaments. This calcium initiates sarcomeric thick and thin filament interraction with consequent sarcomeric shortening. Calcium entry to the cell's contractile machinery continues as long as the membrane remains depolarized. The sarcoplasmic reticulum, stimulated by the increasingly high concentraction of calcium in the area of the underlying sarcomere, begins to pump the cation away from the myofilaments, interraction between the thick and thin sarcomeric components stops, and relaxation occurs (Table 1).

Cell Maintenance and the Production of Energy: The Nucleus and the Mitochondrion

The other principal components of the myofiber, the *nucleus* and its associated systems and the *mitochondria*, are largely concerned with cell maintenance and with the production of high energy compounds necessary for cell work.

The single *nucleus* of the myofiber is located in the center of the cell (Figure 1). It contains the genetic information which allows the cell to construct the new components required for growth, maintenance and repair. Ribonucleic acid, coded by nuclear desoxyribonucleic acid, is exported from the nucleus, probably via the nuclear-cytoplasmic bridges called nuclear pores. It is transported to areas of the cell which require new components via a tubular system called the endoplasmic reticulum. The ribosomes are lined up upon the outer aspect of the endoplasmic reticular membrane, forming the so called rough endoplasmic reticulum and, it is presumed, are transported along these tubular channels to areas of the sarcoplasm where they instruct the formation of new cellular components. Rough endoplasmic reticulum (RER), then, is the hallmark of a cell actively producing new protein, whether it is to be utilized for growth and repair or for export from the cell.

The *mitochondria* lie between the myofibrils, in intimate contact with the sarcomeres, and are also grouped in large pools at either end of the nucleus (Figures 1, 2). They are elliptical bodies containing a complex inner system of membranes arranged in closely packed leaflets called cristae. On these cristae are most of the elements necessary for oxidative phosphorylation and the production of high energy compounds necessary for contractile work and the other energy-consuming processes in the myofiber.

In the following chapters, we will discuss each of the subcellular systems of the myofiber in detail, outlining current concepts of how each functions to produce and sustain the activity of the cardiac cell.

Figure 2. *This is a portion of an ordinary working ventricular cell which shows the components of the myofiber in detail. Note that the thick and thin myofilaments, which make up the sarcomere, are arranged in cylindrical bundles called myofibrils. The myofibrils, separated from one another only by mitochondria and the transverse tubular network, are wrapped into a compact mass by the sarcolemma to form the myofiber, or cardiac cell.*

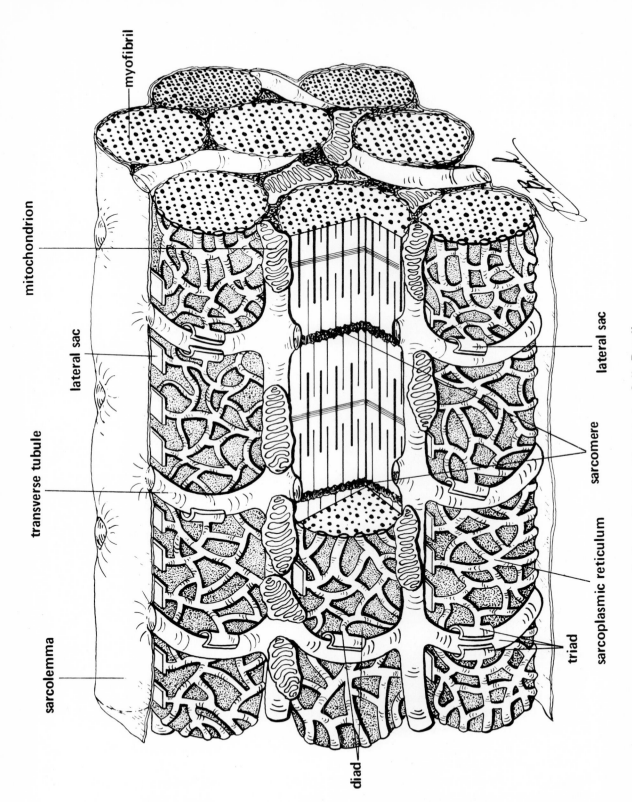

myofibril

mitochondrion

lateral sac

transverse tubule

sarcolemma

diad

triad

sarcoplasmic reticulum

sarcomere

lateral sac

Ordinary Working Ventricular Cell: Detail.

TABLE 1

FUNCTION OF SUBCELLULAR SYSTEMS IN THE MYOFIBER

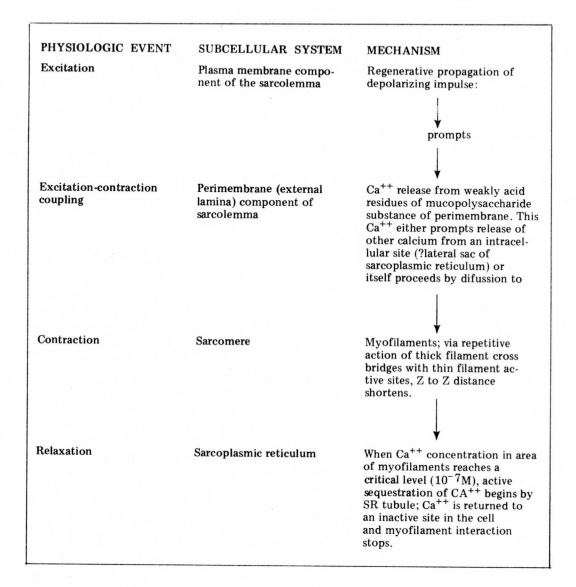

PHYSIOLOGIC EVENT	SUBCELLULAR SYSTEM	MECHANISM
Excitation	Plasma membrane component of the sarcolemma	Regenerative propagation of depolarizing impulse: prompts
Excitation-contraction coupling	Perimembrane (external lamina) component of sarcolemma	Ca^{++} release from weakly acid residues of mucopolysaccharide substance of perimembrane. This Ca^{++} either prompts release of other calcium from an intracellular site (?lateral sac of sarcoplasmic reticulum) or itself proceeds by difussion to
Contraction	Sarcomere	Myofilaments; via repetitive action of thick filament cross bridges with thin filament active sites, Z to Z distance shortens.
Relaxation	Sarcoplasmic reticulum	When Ca^{++} concentration in area of myofilaments reaches a critical level $(10^{-7}M)$, active sequestration of CA^{++} begins by SR tubule; Ca^{++} is returned to an inactive site in the cell and myofilament interaction stops.

General References

Needham, D. M.: *Machina Carnis*. The Biochemistry of Muscular Contraction in its Historical Development. Cambridge University Press. London, 1971.

Legato, M. J.: The Correlation of Ultrastructure and Function in the Mammalian Myocardial Cell. *Prog. Cardiovas. Dis.*, 11:391, 1969.

Legato, M. J.: The Myocardial Cell: New Concepts for the Clinical Cardiologist. *Circ.*, 45:731, 1972.

Legato, M. J.: New Concepts of Cardiac Cellular Structure and Function in *Pathobiology Annual 1972*. Harry L. Ioachim, Ed. Appleton—Century Crofts.: New York, 1972.

CHAPTER II

The Sarcolemma and its Derivatives:
The Transverse Tubular System
and the Intercalated Disc.

The cell membrane is structurally and functionally a complex and sophisticated barrier between the contents of the myofiber and the external environment. It is a dynamic rather than static structure and has many functions. By a combination of active pumping and selective permeability to charged particles, it maintains the ionic dysequilibrium across the cell which is responsible for the resting potential of the myofiber. It supports the process of excitation; its permeability characteristics change in a selective, orderly and predictable sequence which allows specific ions to flow down their electrical and concentration gradients, producing a sequence of changes in the electromotive force across the sarcolemma known collectively as the action potential. It also probably couples excitation to contraction: at the depolarizing signal, a calcium-containing portion of the membrane releases this cation to the area of the myofilaments and interaction between the sarcomeric components begins. It alters the duration of depolarization in response to the frequency of stimulation and, since it continues to release calcium to the area of the myofilaments for as long as the action potential lasts, it is one of the cell components which controls the degree of systolic force the cell generates. Finally, it restores the internal ionic composition of the myofiber to its original state by actively pumping ions (principally sodium) out of the cell at the end of the action potential. In spontaneously depolarizing cells, it is the sarcolemma which, by time and voltage dependent changes in permeability, allows ionic redistribution across the membrane until the potential comes to a level at which the changes in permeability initiating the action potential occur.

The cell membrane, then, sustains excitation, couples excitation to contraction, is one of the determinants of the degree of contractile force generated at each beat of the cell, restores the myofiber to resting equilibrium so that it can be stimulated again and is the component of the myofiber responsible for spontaneous beating in pacemaking cells.

The sarcolemmae of atrial, ventricular and Purkinje cells each generates a unique and characteristic action potential. This implies a functional and probably a structural difference between them. It is very possible, in spite of the rather universally held contention that all membranes have the same fundamental lipoprotein structure (the so-called "unit membrane" theory) that membrane molecular structure is unique for each type of myocardial cell. At its present level of sophistication, the electron microscope cannot be expected to reveal architectural variation between the sarcolemmae of different myofibers, nor does it do so. Indeed, because of the limitations of present techniques, we have a very incomplete knowledge of even what specific ions are carried across the cell membrane and in what concen-

11

trations during excitation and the return to the resting state. There is, however, good evidence that different ions carry the inward and outward currents responsible for the generation of the action potentials of, for example, the Purkinje cell and the ordinary working ventricular cell (1). To a very real extent, then, the physiology of the myofiber is determined by the composition and properties of its delimiting membrane. For this reason, the sarcolemma and its derivatives in the cell deserve detailed discussion.

The Sarcolemma

The delimiting membrane of the myofiber, the sarcolemma, has two parts: the plasma membrane, which appears on the electron micrograph as a thin, electron dense line and the amorphous, granular-appearing basement membrane (also called the perimembrane, or external lamina) which is 5-10 (about 500Å) times thicker than the plasma membrane and is the outermost coating of the myofiber (Figure 1).

The Perimembrane

Strictly speaking, the perimembrane is not a membrane at all: it has no ordered substructure and is an amorphous accumulation at the cell surface of a carbohydrate substance, probably a mucopolysaccharide. Ultrastructurally, it consists of a dense thatchwork of fine filaments embedded in an amorphous, granular material. Langer has offered the concept of the perimembrane as a cation exchange resin, with graded affinities for charged particles such as sodium and calcium. As he has demonstrated in his elegant studies with the electron-dense cation, lanthanum, the probable rôle of the perimembrane is to release calcium ion in response to excitation; the calcium so released penetrates the myofiber and, either directly or indirectly, prompts interraction between thick and thin filaments which effects sarcomeric shortening. We do not know whether perimembrane calcium itself directly engenders myofilament interaction, or whether it releases calcium from an internal storage site which in turn is released to the sarcomere. In any case, it is perimembrane calcium that couples excitation to contraction: if calcium in this portion of the sarcolemma is replaced by another cation (such as lanthanum) the cell is uncoupled: an action potential is generated, but no contraction is evoked. If lanthanum-treated tissue is viewed in the electron microscope, lanthanum is seen bound exclusively to the perimembrane, where presumably it replaced calcium, and in so doing, uncoupled the cell (2).

Calcium is the direct determinant of systolic force developed by the cell: It controls the *degree* to which thick and thin filaments interact: the AMOUNT of calcium released to the sarcomere at the moment of depolarization, as well as the DURATION OF TIME over which the calcium release continues (which is directly proportional to the length of the action potential) determine the number of cross bridges formed between thick and thin filaments and therefore the degree of sarcomeric shortening. *The sarcomere, far from regulating the amount of total cell shortening, is actually a passive agent of the calcium released to it with each depolarization of the cell membrane.* Not only is this cation necessary for the initiation of thick and thin filament interaction, but the total amount presented regulates absolutely the extent of such interaction.

The concept of the perimembrane as a cation exchange resin explains the enhanced contractility of cardiac muscle by low sodium or high calcium ion concentrations in the external environment (3). The negatively charged sites of the perimembrane can be competitively occupied by either sodium or calcium ion: lowering the sodium or increasing the calcium available will both increase the amount of calcium bound by the perimembrane and hence the amount released at the moment of depolarization.

The Plasma Membrane

It is the plasma membrane of the myofiber, the 200Å thick, electron-dense component of the sarcolemma, which sustains the processes of regenerative depolarization and repolarization, contains the machinery for active transport of substances across the cell wall and is the primary component of the semi-permeable barrier between the myofiber and the extracellular space.

Until the past decade, it was widely accepted that all membranes have an identical composition: that they were essentially a bimolecular phospholipid layer, arranged with the non-polar portions of the molecule directed interiorly and the polar heads projecting outward. This layer was sandwiched between two monolayers of protein molecules bound by ionic forces to the charged heads of the lipid moieties. This so-called unit membrane theory has been seriously challenged by good evidence which, taken as a whole, suggests that there is no uniformly applicable model of membrane structure: membranes differ widely in their composition and function. It is difficult, moreover, to attribute all the complex functions they perform to two separated monolayers of protein. More recent models postulate a much higher protein content than has been supposed previously, and a wide variation in both the type and arrangement of such proteins in the membranes of different cells. Such models also stress the fact that the lipid components of the membrane are not the exclusive determinants of protein alignment and therefore of membrane architecture and function, but may only separate the protein-containing subunits of the membrane by adhering to them on two (opposite) sides, allowing them to form a continuous monolayer. The membrane can be asymmetric with respect to some or all of its remaining free sides (potentially a maximum of four, if the protein subunit is envisioned as a cube, for example). Structural asymmetry is essential to many currently postulated theories of membrane function, as we shall see later in our discussion.

Whatever its composition and architecture, the plasma membrane should not be thought of as a static structure; its configuration changes so that the permeability to different ionic species alters cyclically; for example, during the process of excitation, when an inrush of cations (principally sodium) alters the charge across the layer and the cell is activated. Similarly, for example, a change in membrane structure has been involved to explain the active extrusion of sodium from the cell during the restoration of resting ionic equilibrium, wherein the carrier molecule, binding sodium at the interior of the cell and potassium at the outside of the cell, turns 180 degrees within the membrane, thus extruding sodium and carrying potassium in exchange into the cytoplasm (4). The concept of membrane asymmetry with resultant important differences in ion-binding capacity on its inner and outer surfaces and the idea that membrane structure is not fixed and rigid, but cyclically changing, are useful in the explanation of currently known facts about cellular physiology.

Figure 1. *This micrograph is a high power view of the sarcolemma, showing the thin, electron-dense trilaminar plasma membrane (Pl) and the dense thatch work of filaments embedded in amorphous granular material which is called the perimembrane (Pm) or external lamina. ECS = extracellular space. (x 61,600).*

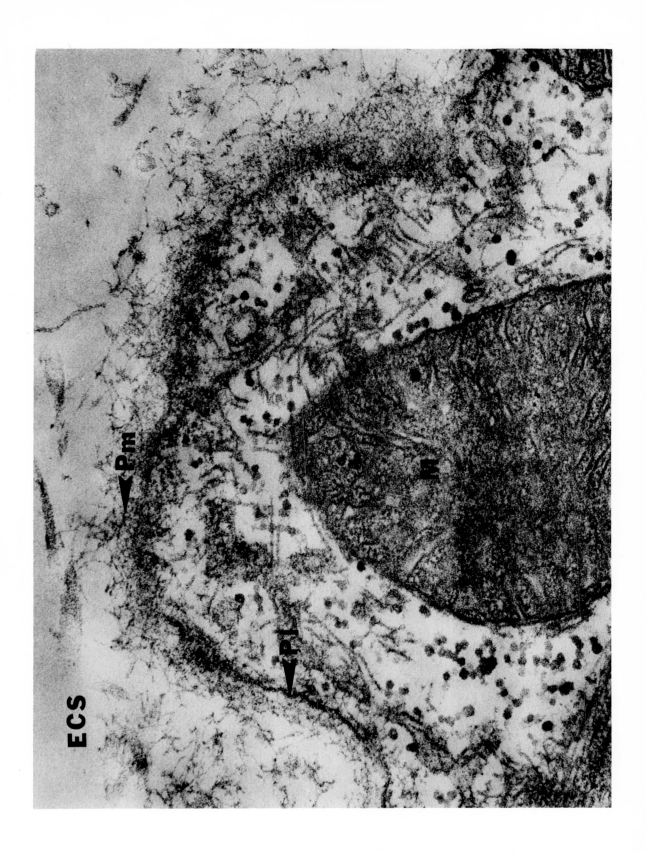

The Action Potential

The plasma membrane of the sarcolemma is a highly organized and precisely structured barrier between the sarcoplasm and the extracellular compartment. By a combination of its permeability characteristics, which prevent the unrestricted diffusion of charged particles across the membrane and by active transport of ions in and/or out of the cell, the membrane maintains a distinct and characteristic difference between the composition of the cytoplasm and the extracellular space. As a result, there is an electrical potential difference across the sarcolemma in the resting state. This potential difference is constant, moreover, implying that there is a balanced ingress and egress of certain ions across the cell wall and no migration at all of others.

When the membrane is stimulated by an exciting impulse, a sequence of time and voltage dependent changes in membrane permeability occurs and allows ions to migrate across the membrane down their electrochemical gradient, thus generating a series of changes in transmembrane potential which occur over a period of about 300 milliseconds and which are collectively termed the "action potential" of the cell. An exciting impulse is one which is strong enough to produce a voltage change in the membrane sufficient to induce a permeability change that allows one (or more) ions to flow across the cell wall. Each migrating ion, by its nature as a charge particle, in turn carries current across the membrane, producing further changes in permeability. Some of these changes are time dependent as well as voltage dependent. Some are *only* time dependent and do not alter at all with voltage. (This accounts, for example, for the long period of the cardiac cell action potential called the "plateau" during which there is no change in net voltage across the membrane, but permeability changes continue to occur, especially with respect to potassium.) *The action potential, then, once initiated, is self-generating and must proceed to completion.*

It is difficult to determine what ions migrate to produce the action potential in cardiac cells. The methods for determining experimentally which ions move across the membrane during an action potential involve the process known as "voltage clamping". In this technique, electrical current passed through the membrane changes the transmembrane potential and holds it at a constant new value. This voltage change, of course, alters membrane permeability (which is a function of transmembrane potential) and ions begin to migrate across the cell wall. Any charged particle crossing the membrane at the new voltage generates a current. Such current is measurable, since it must be opposed to keep the membrane potential constant. Then, by varying the ionic concentration of the solution bathing the membrane, one can dissect out which ions are carrying the measured current at the experimental potential. The nature of the cardiac cell, with its frequent branching and electrically low resistance intercellular connections makes successful clamping very difficult by current methods. What ions actually move in and out of the cell at any given moment during the inscription of the action potential in the myofiber of the mammalian heart is not, therefore, absolutely certain; actually, there are probably complex and simultaneous changes in the distribution of several ions across the sarcolemma during some portions of the action potential. The situation is further complicated by the fact that as the ions migrate, they are influenced by the charge in the membrane itself as well as by the charge on other concomitantly moving ions. Further, the possibility of an opposite and equally charged carrier transporting the ion across the membrane may allow transport without the generation of current. It has even been suggested that injury to the cell membrane may change the identity of the ions that migrate at any given moment during the excitatory process; the transmembrane migration of quite different ions may be responsible for the generation of the same phases of the action potential in the cell when it has sustained membrane damage as compared to when it is healthy.

The shape of the action potential varies among the various types of myofibers: atrial, ventricular and Purkinje cells all have characteristic and different action potentials by which they can be identified. There is good evidence, moreover, that different ions carry the inward and outward currents in different cardiac cell species, inferring that membrane molecular structure and therefore its permeability characteristics are unique for any given type of cell in the heart (1).

Whatever the composition of the cell membrane, and whatever the shape, it is generally agreed that the action potential can be divided into five phases, 0 through 4. The data concerning which ions move across the membrane which we will summarize, are a composite that can be considered generally applicable to the majority of cardiac cells.

At the exciting signal, membrane permeability to sodium changes abruptly, sodium rushes into the cell from the extracellular compartment and raises the interior of the cell from -90mV to +20mV, a total of 110mV change in transmembrane potential. This is *phase 0* of the action potential (Figure 2). The actual amount of sodium influx has been quantitated by isotopic studies, and amounts to about $13\mu\mu M/cm^2$ of membrane (3). The sodium inrush reverses the sign across the membrane so that the interior of the cell is now positive with respect to the exterior. A certain amount of inward current is carried by calcium ion; exactly how much is not known, but Niedergerke suggests that, at least in Purkinje fiber, the last portion of phase 0, the so-called "overshoot", is carried by calcium ion (5).

Phase 1, a small return of the membrane towards repolarization, is probably due to an egress of chloride ion from the cell.

Phase 2 is a most interesting portion of the action potential. More than one ionic species is migrating simultaneously during this time, although the potential across the membrane is held at an almost constant level. This phase of the action potential is dominated by slow, gradual change in permeability to sodium (gNa) (g=membrane conductance, or the ability of the membrane to allow ionic migration at a given voltage across it). The high gNa declines very slowly, and a total of $64\mu\mu M/cm^2$ inward flux of Na^+ (almost ten times the resting membrane Na^+ flux) helps to maintain the cell at this level of depolarization. The total flux of sodium across the membrane to the end of the plateau is $64\mu\mu+13\mu\mu$ or $77\mu\mu M/cm^2$, almost 13 times the resting flux of Na^+; such flux requires 2-2.5% of cardiac energy (3).

There is also a slow inward calcium current during the action potential plateau. As membrane gNa declines, gK, the conductivity of the membrane to potassium slowly rises. This slow and late change in the ability of the membrane to allow K^+ to leave the cell is called *delayed rectification*: in some instances, the gK is even less than it is at resting membrane potential; this is termed *anomalous rectification*. The plateau is terminated by a sudden increase in membrane permeability to potassium, and a sudden, rapid efflux of K^+ from the interior of the cell to the outside restores the cell to resting potential. This produces phase 3 of the action potential, a sudden drop of transmembrane potential from a high to a resting value.

Calcium depletion of the sarcolemma with excitation has been invoked to

Figure 2. *These sketches represent phases 0 through 4 of the action potential. The important changes in ionic redistribution across the membrane during phases 0-4 are indicated.*

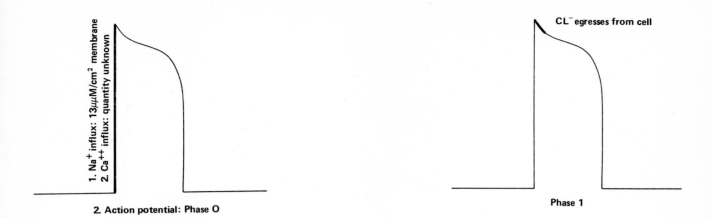

1. Na^+ influx: $13\mu\mu M/cm^2$ membrane
2. Ca^{++} influx: quantity unknown

2. Action potential: Phase O

CL^- egresses from cell

Phase 1

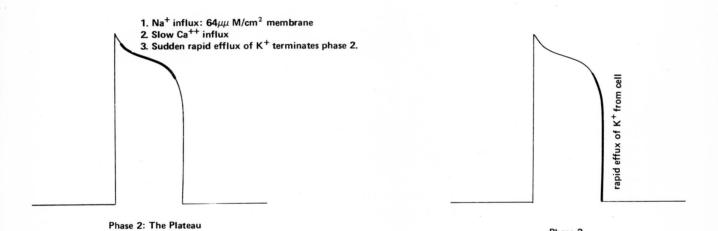

1. Na^+ influx: $64\mu\mu$ M/cm^2 membrane
2. Slow Ca^{++} influx
3. Sudden rapid efflux of K^+ terminates phase 2.

Phase 2: The Plateau

rapid effux of K^+ from cell

Phase 3.

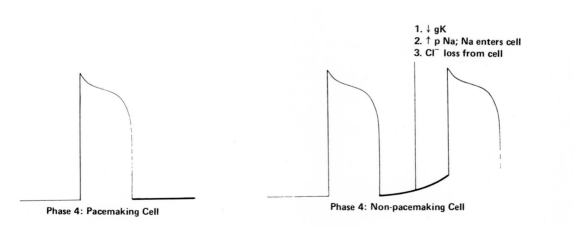

1. ↓ gK
2. ↑ p Na; Na enters cell
3. Cl^- loss from cell

Phase 4: Pacemaking Cell

Phase 4: Non-pacemaking Cell

Phase 4: Na^+-K^+ exchange via operation of sodium pump

explain the persistence of a low gK during the plateau; replacement of membrane calcium is thought to mediate the increase in gK that terminates the plateau and initiates *phase 3* of the action potential.

At the beginning of *phase 4* the cell, although at a normal resting potential, is rich in sodium and poor in potassium. The membrane sodium pump, stimulated by the increase in internal Na^+ concentration inside the cell, begins to extrude Na^+ from the cell, and pull in K^+ from the extracellular space in a cationic exchange that keeps the transmembrane potential constant while restoring the cell's internal composition to the Na^+-poor, K^+-rich mixture. Opit and Charnok envision the Na^+ pump working via a carrier molecule in the membrane which attaches Na^+ at the interior of the cell and K^+ at the outer membrane surface, turns 180° within the membrane, and extrudes Na^+ to the exterior, while bringing in K^+ ion (4). Such a procedure, of course, consumes energy and is called, therefore, an active process.

There are four factors controlling the activity of the sodium pump: the change in membrane potential, the decreased amount of membrane calcium, the increase in concentration of Na^+ at the interior of the cell and the accumulation of K^+ at the exterior surface of the membrane. The "membrane ATPase", as the Na^+ pump is sometimes called, then, is responsive to a whole constellation of factors in the environment of the membrane itself and the solutions on either side of it.

We know that there are ions, specifically Na^+ and K^+, which cross the cell even at rest.

In cells which do not pace themselves (i. e., spontaneously reach threshold and depolarize) during the resting phase there is a constant small Na^+ flux ($5.9\mu\mu M/cm^2/sec$) due to a rather low permeability of the membrane to Na^+ at resting levels (3). Sodium, which tends to flow down its concentration gradient from the extracellular compartment, where its concentration is 143mM to the interior of the cell, where its concentration is 27-30mM, crosses the cell by passive diffusion via a membrane carrier; intracellular Na^+ concentration is kept low with reference to the extracellular compartment by active extrusion of sodium from the cell.

In contrast to the low pNa of the myofiber at rest, membrane pK is much higher, and K^+ flux during rest in non-pacemaking cells is measured anywhere from 1.5-$5xNa^+$ flux, ($3\mu\mu M$-$19\mu\mu$moles cm^2/sec K^+ flux). The much greater K^+ flux with respect to Na^+ flux, as Langer has pointed out, indicates that Na^+-K^+ exchange is not interrelated on a 1:1 basis (3).

In pacemaker cells the picture is different and rather more complex: there is a time and voltage-dependent fall in membrane conductivity to K^+ (gK) and a late increase in Na^+ permeability near threshold which is also voltage dependent (gNa). As gK diminishes, chloride flows out of the cell. All of these changes in permeability allow the passage of ions across the membrane, the membrane potential rises to threshold and an action potential is generated.

The problem of refractoriness is a difficult one to explain; it is probable that membrane is affected by a current, no matter at what stage during the action potential it is applied. Hoffman and Cranefield, aware of this fact, define the effective refractory period as one in which an electrical stimulus, no matter how strong, does not induce a propogated action potential in cardiac tissue and feels that this period lasts until the end of the plateau or phase 2, of the action potential. There follows the relative refractory period, which begins with the time when a strong stimulus (albeit followed by an abnormally long latent period) evokes a propogated action potential. This is immediately followed by the so-called supernormal period, during which the cell can be stimulated with more ease than during in its resting state. The supernormal period is brief, and is over by the early part of phase 4.

The Transverse Tubular System

The transverse tubular system is a sarcolemmal derivative and both components of the cell wall, the perimembrane and the plasma membrane, participate in its formation. The plasma membrane of the sarcolemma is contiguous with and forms the walls of the transverse tubular system as it extends downward from the cell surface to honeycomb the interior of the myofiber in a system of channels open to the extracellular compartment. The T-system lumen is filled with the amorphous, granular-appearing substance of the perimembrane (Figure 3).

Simply on the basis of the details of the architecture of transverse tubular system, ideas of T-tubular function have gradually taken shape, none of which are, in the light of the most current evidence, likely to be correct. First, since the T-system lumen is anatomically open to and continuous with the extracellular compartment at the surface of the myofiber, it was thought that the extracellular space was essentially present *in a completely unmodified way* at virtually all levels of the myofiber. Second, because of the proximity of the T-system to the calcium depots of the lateral sacs of the sarcoplasmic reticulum, the triad or diad was postulated to be the anatomic substrate for the coupling of excitation to contraction. The depolarizing impulse, passing in an uninterrupted and unaltered fashion over the sarcolemma, was thought to effect calcium release from the lateral sac to the area of the myofilaments, where it prompted interaction between the thick and thin filaments and initiated the contractile event.

There is histochemical evidence that the perimembrane in the transverse tubular lumen may not have a composition identical to that at the cell surface: although fundamentally the perimembrane in the T-tubular lumen is the same as that of the sarcolemma: a carbohydrate with weakly acid residues. Howse has shown that reuthenium red, which stains the perimembrane at the cell surface does not attach at all to the lamina filling the T-tubular lumen in mammalian myocardium (6). He also points out that although the external lamina of the sarcolemma has nucleoside monophosphatase activity, the transverse tubular lumen does not.

There is further indirect evidence to suggest that the transverse tubular lumen does not always have the same ionic composition as the extracellular space; if myocardium is perfused with chloride-poor perfusate, the tissue viewed in the electron microscope shows a specific dilatation of the transverse tubules, suggesting that Cl^- ion diffuses from the cell into the Cl^- poor milieu of the T-tubular lumen, is bound there, at least transiently, and thus prevented from rapid equilibration with the contents of the extracellular space at the surface of the cell (7). A hyperosmotic environment is thus created and water is drawn into the T-tubular space, specifically dilating that compartment of the myofiber. Similarly, the persistent afterpotential in muscle following a rapid train of stimuli might be on the basis of the binding of the K^+ leaving the stimulated cell to a substance in the T-tubule, probably the weakly acid residues of the perimembrane. Charged particles coming from the sarcoplasm into the lumen of the extracellular space

21

Figure 3. *In this electron micrograph, the extracellular space (ECS) is marked by the electron-dense salt, sodium antimonate (NaSb). The precipitate passes down into the depth of the cell via the lumen of the transverse tubule (T) which is a sarcolemmal derivative. M = mitochondrion (x 49,000).*

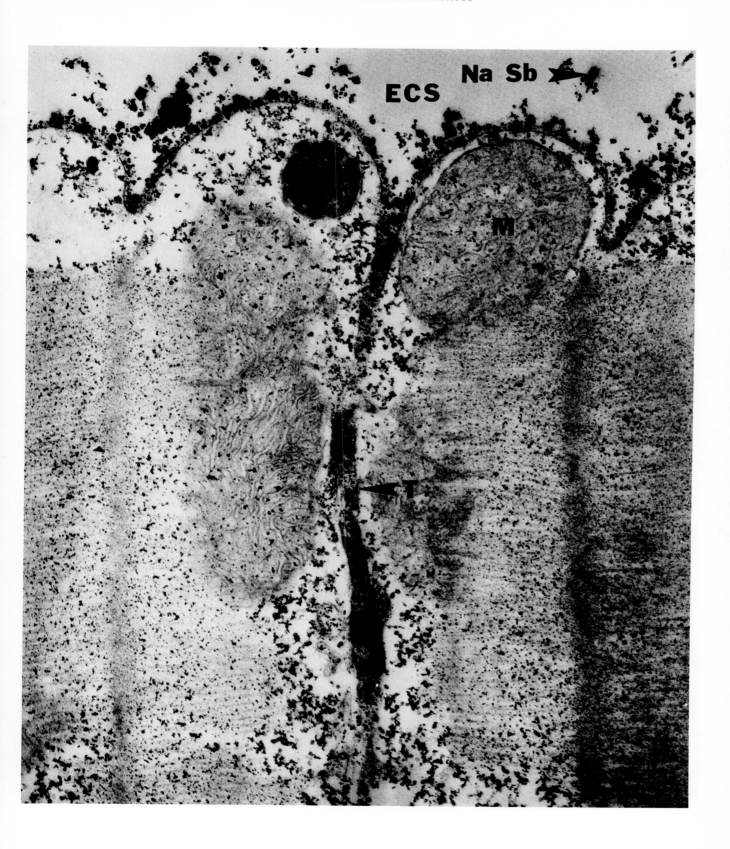

probably cannot, because of the nature and properties of the perimembrane, equilibrate rapidly or in an unrestricted fashion with the extracellular compartment at the surface of the cell. It is likely, then, that the composition of the contents of the transverse tubular system and the extracellular compartment are really different and perhaps significantly so.

The cell with a transverse tubular system, then, becomes potentially a very different cell from those myofibers which have one (like the great majority of atrial and Purkinje cells, for example). Localized build ups of cations, such as potassium, in the T-lumen are probable, and become more important as the rate of cell beating increases and less time is available between cycles for the equilibration of the contents of the T-tubular lumen with the extracellular milieu at the cell surface. This has fundamentally important implications in the functional properties of the cell, especially those which are related to the membrane. For example, the shape and duration of the action potential and even, perhaps, whether the cell is excitable at all (by virtue of a change in potential which is the consequence of ionic build up, however transient, in the transverse tubular lumen) may be related to the presence or absence of this system in the cell.

If the T-tubular system is not a vehicle for the unmodified extension of the extracellular compartment throughout the body of the myofiber, neither is it a prerequisite for excitation-contraction coupling in the myocardial cell. The ordinary working ventricular cell is the only one of the three principal types of myofibers to have a transverse tubular system: the great majority of atrial and Purkinje cells do not have one. Yet all three types beat, and beat synchronously. Moreover, ventricular cells grown in tissue culture do not develop a T-system until long after they have been synchronously beating at rates as high as 180. The primitive myoblast is self-pacing. This ability is lost as the cell grows and differentiates. It may be that the development of a transverse tubular system extinguishes the ability of the cell to depolarize spontaneously. As Hoffman and Cranefield point out, the pacemaking cells in the adult ventricular myocardium are not the ventricular working cells, (which have a T system) but Purkinje fibers, in which this subcellular system is conspicuously absent.

Intercellular Connections: The Intercalated Disc

Cardiac cells beat in a virtually simultaneous fashion: one cell, depolarizing at a faster rate than any of the others, can capture the entire population of the heart. This implies that there is essentially no interference with the transmission of impulses from cell to cell, and means that an action potential generated in one myofiber is propagated without significant delay to neighboring cells through electrically low resistance junctions.

Anatomically, cardiac cells make contact with one another in a variety of ways. These vary in complexity from a simple intermingling of the external laminae (perimembranes) of closely approximated myofibers to the extensive, highly specialized and intricate intercellular link peculiar to cardiac tissue called *the intercalated disc* (Figure 4). The pattern and extent of connection between myofibers varies with the type of cells in the heart and often, as we will see in the chapters dealing with the specific ultrastructure of atrial, ventricular and Purkinje tissue, can be correlated to some extent with the distinctive electrical properties of different types of myofibers.

The intercalated disc, like the transverse tubular system, is a sarcolemmal derivative and is formed by the plasma and perimembranes of adjacent myfibers. From an anatomic point of view, it has four divisions. The simplest, called the "unspecialized" or "intermediate" portion, lies parallel to the long axis of the cell between the two myofibers. The remaining three portions of the disc, the fascia adherens, the nexus and the desmosome, are ultrastructurally more complex. The *fascia adherens* is the portion of the disc separating the terminal sarcomeres of adjoining cells: under the sarcolemma on either side of the extracellular space is an accumulation of Z substance which is thicker, more irregular in shape and anatomically less organized than the sarcolemmal Z band but into which the thin filaments of the terminal sarcomere insert.

The two most specialized areas of the disc are the desmosomal and the nexal portions. Both are anatomically very complex and serve as firm sites of attachment between cells and/or, possibly, as the junction across which efficient impulse transmission can occur.

The *desmosome* is a multi-layered complex about $0/5\mu$ in diameter in which the gap between the adjacent cells measures 250-300Å (Figure 5). Sjöstrand pointed out that this apparent space is bisected by a thin, electron-dense line, and that there are cross bridges at right angles to this line connecting it to the sarcolemmae on either side of the intercellular gap (8). Rayns and Simpson, who labelled the extracellular space enclosed by the intercalated disc with lanthanum, showed that, as Sjöstrand had suggested, the apparent gap between cells has a highly ordered ultrastructure (9). They postulate that the thin, electron-dense line bisecting the intercellular space in the desmosome is the mucopolysaccharide of the conjoined perimembranes of the adjacent cells, and that the cross bridges serve to keep the diameter of the gap constant and give rigidity to the configuration.

With the advent of electron microscopy, investigators were able to probe the ultrastructure of the *nexal portion* of the intercalated disc for the first time (Figure 6). Initially it was felt by most anatomists that there was a gap between cells at the nexal junction or at the most, a fusion of the outer membrane leaflets of adjacent cells. The myocardium, it was said, acted as if it were a continuous sheet of tissue but the general feeling was that there was no actual structural bridge between myofibers.

We owe the best analysis of the architecture of the nexal portion of the intercalated disc to McNutt (10). His elegant studies of freeze-cleaved cells fractured through their nexal junctions have resulted in an elaborate model which presents the nexus not as the simple apposition or fusion of sarcolemmae of adjacent cells, but as a place in the intercalated disc which is honeycombed by a system of cross-connections between cells. He envisions these channels as bridges between cells and although he does not flatly state that there is continuity of the sarcoplasm from one myofiber to another, he implies that these are "direct routes" for intercellular communication. He estimates their diameter to be 15-20Å and points out that ions might certainly pass through such a system of "hydrophilic channels". With the work of McNutt, then, we have come once again to the idea that cardiac tissue may be an anatomic as well as a functional syncitium: myofibers may actually have cytoplasmic channels which form a continuum from one cell to another at the nexal junctions.

There are isolated desmosomal links between cells in the heart as well along the course of the specialized portions of the intercalated disc. It is tempting to

Figure 4. *This is an electron micrograph of an intercalated disc (arrows) which joins two myocardial cells. N = nexus. D = Desmosome. FA = fascia adherens. NSP = non-specialized portion. ECS = extracellular space. Pm = perimembrane. Pl = plasma membrance. S = sarcomere. M = mitochondrion. G = glycogen granules. (x 26,000).*

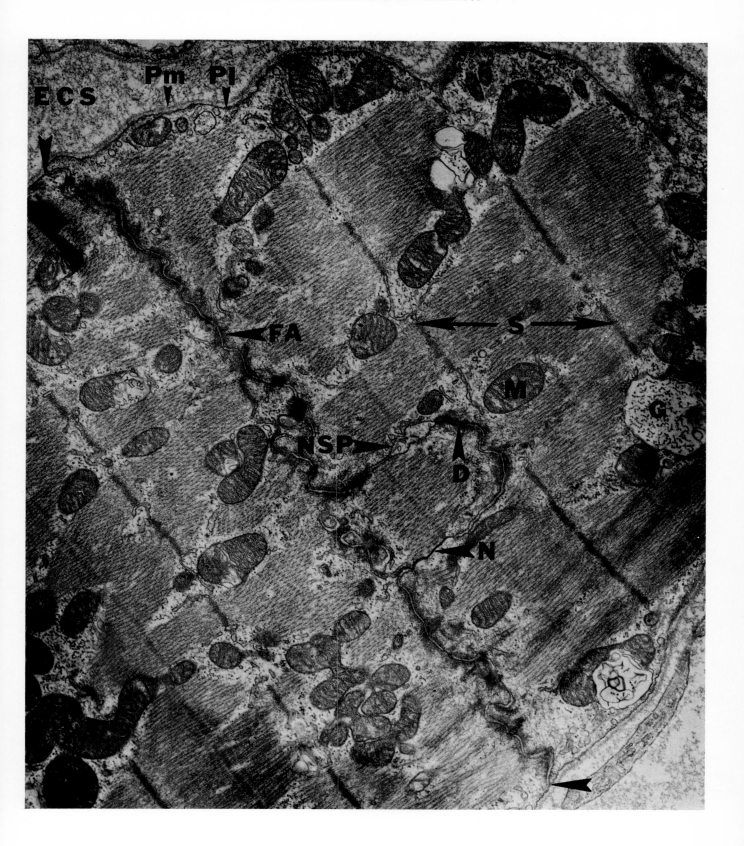

Figure 5. *This is a micrograph of the desmosome, the specialized link between cells. It is multi-layered. What appears at this magnification to be the central single line of the structure (arrows) is actually a gap between cells which has a highly ordered ultrastructure (see text). (x 68,155).*

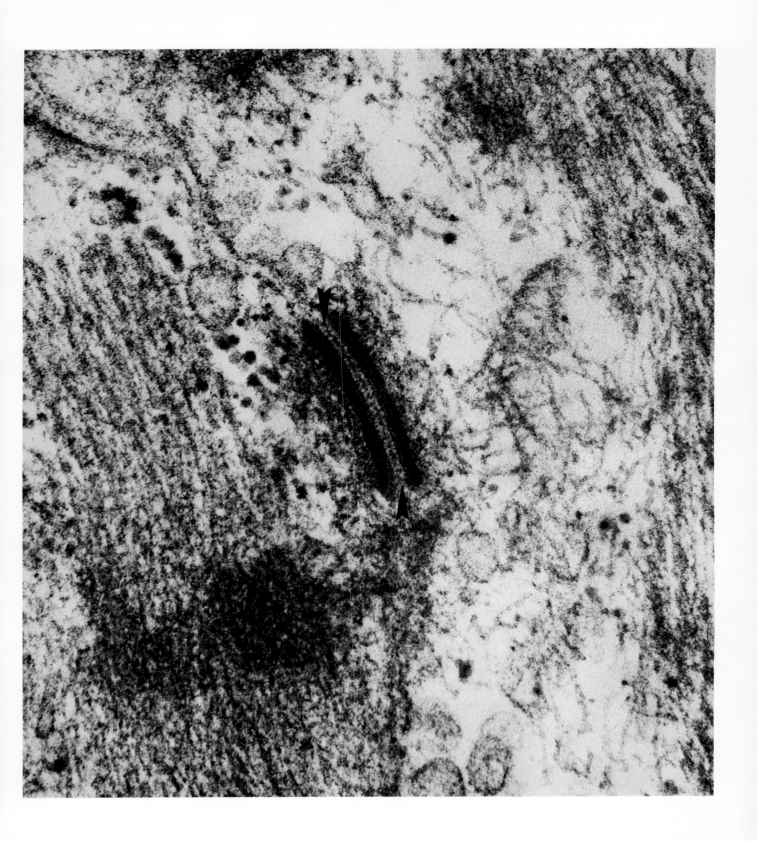

Figure 6. *In the nexal junction, the sarcolemmae of adjacent cells are closely apposed, but not actually fused. Note the cross-linkages between cells within the nexus at right angles to the long axis of the junction (circle). These are said to be actual cytoplasmic bridges between cells (see text). (x 208,125).*

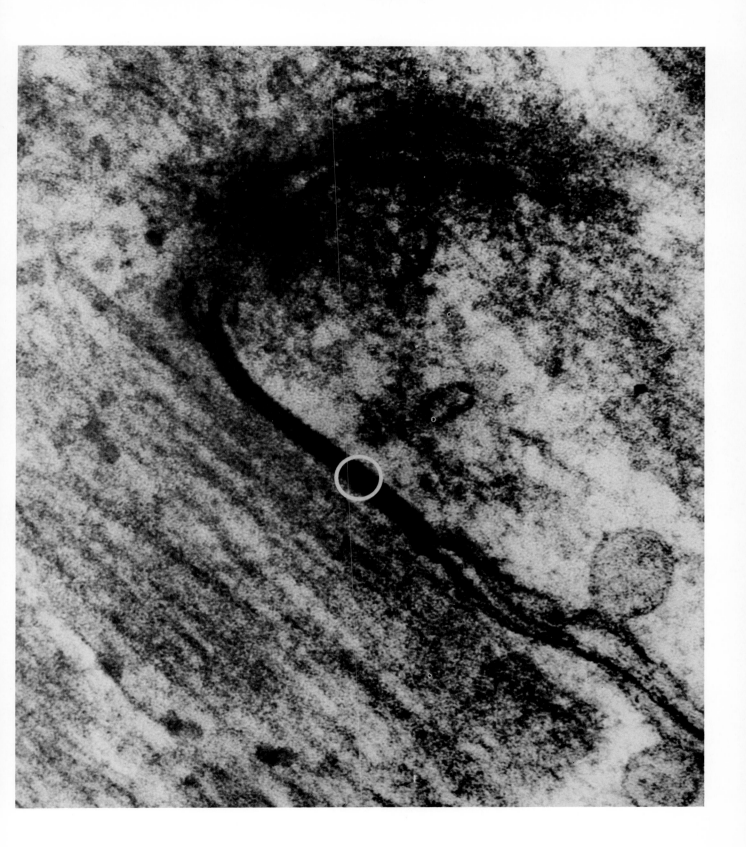

postulate that these highly specialized junctions, the nexus and/or the desmosome, whether anatomically they exist by themselves or in the disc, are the low-resistance sites at which impulse transmission between cells is affected. McNutt's model makes the nexal junction seem especially suited to this function (10). There is excellent evidence to suggest, however, that the nexus is not actually essential to intercellular impulse transmission. Sheets of rat ventricular cells grown in tissue culture, for example, beat in unison well before nexal junctions have begun to develop (11). Baldwin, who has destroyed electrical communications between frog atrial cells by mechanical injury, shows that while such treatment injures desmosomes, it leaves nexal junctions anatomically undisturbed, at least ultrastructurally (12). Muir's data shows that calcium depletion destroys desmosomal linkages, but that nexuses are not affected by calcium depletion and emphasizes that there are differences in chemical composition between the two junctions (13). Jewett and his colleagues offer the observation that there are no nexal junctions in chicken embryonal myocardium or in the hearts of young chickens, adding further evidence to support the proposition that nexuses are not required for the synchronized beating of cardiac cells (14).

Kawamura, in his review on intercellular linkages, makes the point that the definitive experiment, in which the nexal linkages between cells is selectively disrupted and the effect on electrical coupling between myofibers observed, has not been done; whatever disrupts nexuses also destroys desmosomal connections and in general, tends to increase the spaces between cells (15).

The function of the nexal junction, then, is not clear. As McNutt points out, its appearance varies with the method of tissue preparation: McNutt interprets this to mean there is one type of nexal junction and that, if it is properly preserved, it will show a gap between the outer leaflets of adjacent sarcolemmae (10), (See Figure 6). Others, like Brightman, maintain that there are nexal junctions in which the membranes of the participating cells are actually fused and that this appearance is not artifactual (16). Brightman who calls such a junction a "tight" junction maintains that both the "tight" and "gap" junctions allow impulse transmission between cells.

In summary, the anatomic evidence for implicating the nexus and, although perhaps to a lesser extent, the desmosome, as sites for electrically low resistance connections between cells is compelling. We do not have any direct evidence, however, which labels the nexus indispensable for, or the only site of, electrical coupling between myofibers. Moreover, there are many species in which myocardial cells beat synchronously without nexuses in a embryonic or young postnatal stage of life.

There are whole populations of cells in the adult heart which have no or only rare nexal junctions: atrial cells have relatively few and the specialized pacing cells (P cells) of the sinus node are without any nexal junctions at all (17). Obviously, then, the nexus is not essential to impulse transmission between cells.

Desmosomal junctions are, in contrast to the nexus, universally present between *all types* of myocardial cells, including ventricular cells grown in tissue culture, where they exist at very early stages of development if only in rudimentary form (18). It may well be that the desmosome is an electrically low resistance connection between myocardial cells and that the number of these specialized linkages between cells is related to the speed of conduction in tissue.

Specific References

1. Miller, J. P., Wallace, A. G., and Feezor, M. D.: A Quantitative Comparison of the Relation between the Shape of the Action Potential and the Pattern of Stimulation in Canine Ventricular Muscle and Purkinje Fibers. *J. Mol. and Cell. Cardiol.* 2:3, 1971.
2. Langer, G. A. and Frank, J. S.: Lanthanum in Heart Cell Culture. Effect on Calcium Exchange Correlated with Its localization. *J. Cell Biol.*, 54:441, 1972.
3. Langer, G. A.: Ion Fluxes in Cardiac Excitation and Contraction and Their Relation to Myocardial Contractility. *Physiol. Rev.*, 48:708, 1968.
4. Opit, L. J. and Charnock, J. S.: A Molecular Model For A Sodium Pump. *Nature*, 208:471, 1965.
5. Niedergerke, R.: Calcium and activation of contraction. *Experientia*, 15:128, 1959.
6. Howse, H. D., Ferrans, V. J., and Hibbs, R. G.: A Comparative Histochemical and Electron Microscopic Study of the Surface Coatings of Cardiac Muscle Cells. *J. Mol. Cell. Cardiol.* 1:57, 1970.
7. Legato, M. J.: Ultrastructural Alterations Produced in Mammalian Myocardium by Variation In Perfusate Ionic Composition. *J. Cell. Biol.*, 31:1, 1968.
8. Sjöstrand, F. S., Anderson—Cedergren, and Dewey, M. M.: The Ultrastructure of the Intercalated Discs of Frog, Mouse and Guinea Pig Cardiac Muscle. *J. Ultrastruct. Res.*, 1:271, 1958.
9. Rayns, D. G., Simpson, J. O., and Ledingham, J. M.: Ultrastructure of Desmosomes in Mammalian Intercalated Disc; Appearances After Lanthanum Treatment. *J. Cell Biol.*, 42:322, 1969.
10. McNutt, N. S. and Weinstein, R. S.: The Ultrastructure of the Nexus. A Correlated Thin Section and Freeze-Cleave Study. *J. Cell. Biol.*, 47:666, 1970.
11. Hararay, I. and Farley, B.: *In vitro* Studies on Single Beating Rat Heart Cells. I. Growth and Organization. *Exp. Cell. Res.*, 29:454, 1963.
12. Baldwin, K. M.: The Fine Structure and Electrophysiology of Heart Muscle Cell Injury. *J. Cell. Biol.*, 46:455, 1970.
13. Muir, A. R.: The Effects of Divalent Cations on the Cellular Structure of Cardiac Muscle. *J. Anat.*, 99:27, 1965.
14. Jewett, P. H., Sommer, J. R., and Johnson, E. A.: Cardiac muscle. Its ultrastructure in the Finch and Hummingbird with Special Reference to the Sarcoplasmic Reticulum. *J. Cell Biol.*, 49:50, 1971.
15. Kawamura, K. and James, T. N.: Comparative Ultrastructure of Cellular Junctions in Working Myocardium and the Conduction System under Normal and Pathologic Conditions. *J. Mol. Cell. Cardiol.*, 3:31, 1971.
16. Brightman, M. W. and Reese, T. S.: Junctions Between Intimately Apposed Cell Membranes in the Vertebrate Brain. *J. Cell. Biol.*, 40:648, 1969.
17. James, T. N., Sherf, L., Fine. G., Morales, A. R.: Comparative Ultrastructure of the Sinus Node in Man and Dog. *Circ.*, 34:139, 1966.
18. Legato, M. J.: Ultrastructural Characteristics of the Rat Ventricular Cell Grown in Tissue Culture, with Special Reference to Sarcomerogenesis. *J. Mol. Cell. Cardiol.*, 4:299, 1972.

General References

Hoffman, F. and Cranefield, P.: *Electrophysiology of the Heart.* McGraw-Hill Book Company, Inc., N. Y., 1960.
Langer, G. A.: Coupling Calcium in Mammalian Ventricle: Its Source and Factors Regulating Its Quantity. *Cardiovas. Res. Supplement*, 1:71, 1971.
Langer, G. A.: The Ionic Basis for Control of Myocardial Contractility. *Prog. Cardiovas. Dis. 9:*194, 1966.

CHAPTER III

The Sarcomere and the Contractile Event

The bulk of the muscle is made up of sarcomeres, the contractile units of the myofiber. They are arranged side-to-side in long rows called myofibrils which in the ordinary working cell run uninterrupted except for the nucleus, from one end of the cell to the other. Essentially, the sarcomere is a cylindrical bundle of two types of filaments or myofilaments, as they are called, one thick and the other thin, which interdigitate with one another and are packed in precise hexagonal patterns (Figures 1, 2, 3). The sarcomere is delimited at either end by the "Z" disc, into which the thinner of the two kinds of filaments insert.

If one cuts through the cell parallel to its long axis (see Fig. 1, Chap. 1), the long rows of sarcomeres are seen as repeating units with a characteristic banded pattern. The thin filaments, embedded in the dark, electron dense Z-band, pass centrally from either end of the sarcomere to interdigitate with a group of thicker and more electron dense filaments occupying the central portion of the contractile unit. These thick filaments make up the "A" band. The lightest portion of the sarcomere, where thin filaments exist alone, and where they do not interdigitate with thick filaments, is called the "I" band.

The letters Z, I and A are not merely arbitrary, but date from the 19th century, when muscle was first examined in microscopes using both ordinary and polarized light. Z comes from the German word "Zwischenscheibe", or "between disc", indicating that the Z structure is a round plate, separating filaments of adjacent sarcomeres. "A" refers to the anisotropic nature of the thick filaments, which are doubly refractile and hence, bright in polarized light, although they appear dark when viewed with the ordinary light microscope. "I" refers to the fact that the thin filaments do not have this property and were thus called isotropic.

It is the interaction between thin and thick filaments that causes sarcomeric shortening. The exact details of how this occurs still elude us; indeed, our information about the exact composition and architecture of the filaments themselves is incomplete, in spite of great advances in the technology of microscopes and tissue preparation that have been made since Leeuwenhock first looked at muscle three centuries ago in 1674 (1). A great deal of incisive work has been done in the last decade due to special techniques of filament isolation and advances in methods of tissue preparation for viewing in the electron microscope, however, and we are beginning to get some insight into how muscle shortens.

The Thin Filament

Many proteins combine to make up the thin filament. The major constituent, however, is the protein actin. G, or globular, actin is a spherical molecule about

55Å (55/10,000 or about 1/200 of a micron, or 1/2,000 of a mm) in diameter (2) and with a molecular weight of about 50,000 (3). In the presence of magnesium, ATP and calcium, G-actin polymerizes into F or fibrous actin, which is a double stranded helix with a pitch of about 365Å: The two linear strands of polymerized G-actin are wound together much like a double strand of beads, one twisted about the other (Figure 3). The double stranded, helical nature of the thin filament with its globular subunits is clearly visible in the electron microscope with properly prepared specimens (4). ATP is split in the polymerization process and ADP, along with a divalent cation, is incorporated into the G-actin molecule. These combinations stabilize the G molecule configuration so that polymerization can occur.

Actin accounts for only 60% of the I-Band protein. There are many more proteins than actin in the thin filament, probably more than have yet been discovered, as a matter of fact, although the electron microscope has not really helped to show their configuration. Even their location in the sarcomere can only be inferred from special studies such as those with labelled antibody preparations.

The final length of the thin filament is 1μ and in living muscle it is never longer. This fixed and constant length is probably due to the action of one of the newly discovered, so called "structural" proteins, β-actinin, which binds to the terminal G-actins on the filament and prevents further addition of subunits (5, 6). It has been suggested that β-actinin may bind to the sides of the thin filaments as well, preventing their entanglement with one another and allowing them to remain at fixed distances from one another in the sarcomere.

The second structural protein is α-actinin, which has three distinct components, identifiable by their different sedimentation characteristics; 6S, 10S, and 25S moities have been isolated. The 6-S component of alpha actinin is found in the Z Band (7). Although the helix of the thin filament is formed by two strands of actin; the filament separates at the Z Band into four strands, which fan out to form the corners of a square, the two anterior legs lying in one plane, and the other two lying posteriorly. Thus in longitudinal section, the thin filament breaks into a Y-shape just before it terminates at the Z disc (Figure 4). The 6-S component of alpha actinin may serve as a cement which fixes the legs of the I filament into the substance of the Z-band; in vitro, actinin causes F-actin to aggregate into amorphous nets. Alpha-actinin has also been found along two seldom noticed lines in the I-Band perpendicular to the long axis of the filaments and parallel to the Z disc. These lines are named N1 and N2 by Franzini—Armstrong, who opines that actinin binds to the thin filaments at these points, even forming fine tufts between them which serve to hold them at rigidly fixed distances from one another near their point of entry into the Z-Band (8). She observes that beyond a certain point a short distance away from the Z band, it seems that the inter-filament distance is no longer rigid; they can be pushed out of position by glycogen particles which are interposed between them. Alpha-actinin, then, may serve to keep the interfilament distance in the I band constant so that their position as they enter the substance of the Z band is precisely correct (5, 6, 8).

The thin filament contains two other proteins which are crucial in the initiation of the contractile event; these are tropomyosin B* and troponin. Tropomyosin is

---

*Tropomyosin B is so called to distinguish it from tropomyosin A, or paramyosin, the protein found in smooth muscles of some invertebrates which allows muscle to develop a prolonged, sustained contraction—the so called "catch" mechanism.

referred to as a "modulatory" protein and, although its role in the sarcomere is unknown, it inhibits magnesium-activated interaction between actin and myosin in vitro.

The troponin complex sits on the thin filament at 400 Å intervals, attached to the strand of tropomyosin which lies in the groove between the two chains of actin monomers (9). Troponin has three separate moieties (10): one component forms the link attaching the troponin complex to tropomyosin, another fragment serves as a calcium receptor, with a single high affinity site for this cation and the third obstructs an unknown number of "active sites" on the thin filament (probably more than one, and perhaps many). If calcium is added to the tropomyosin-troponin complexes, its configuration is changed in such a way that the active sites on the thin filament are exposed and interraction between it and the thick filament ensues.

To summarize, then, actin is the major component of the thin filament. It is only 60% of the total protein in the I filaments, however; there are two structural proteins, α and β-actinin, which regulate the interfilamentous distance as the actin-strands approach the Z disc, cement them firmly into Z substance, and determine their final and constant length of 1μ. There are also the modulatory proteins, tropomyosin and troponin, which govern the interaction between thin and thick filaments.

The Thick Filament

In contrast to the heterogeneous nature of the thin filament, the thick filament is composed almost entirely of a single protein, myosin. The details of the architecture of the myosin molecule and how they are stacked together to make up the thick filament are not completely known, but we have a good working knowledge of the general characteristics of thick filament ultrastructure.

The myosin molecule is essentially a rod ending in a globular head (Figure 5). The head, which is 200 Å tall and 60 Å wide, has enzymatic properties; it splits ATP without being consumed. The rod, which consists of two parallel helically arranged polypeptide chains,* is about 1300 Å long and gives the molecule the strength and rigidity of a fibrous protein. Myosin, therefore, is unique; it has the properties of an enzyme on the one hand and on the other, of a structural protein which can sustain and transmit contractile force.

A great deal of investigation has been devoted to determining the exact structural details of the myosin molecule; its total weight, after all, is 500,000. Different procedures, quite naturally, yield different molecular fragments: proteolytic digestion of the polypeptide chains of myosin results in quite different subunits than does disruption of nonpeptide linkages, such as disulfide bridges or hydrogen bonds.

Urea, which disrupts non-peptide intramolecular bonds, produces two groups of subfragments: a heavy subunit and three or four light subunits (11). It is the latter, which weigh about 20,000, that probably convey ATPase activity on the myosin molecule. The ATPase activity of myosin differs in various types of muscle with the speed at which the muscle must contract. Such variations are probably the consequence of differences in the structure of these light chains or

---

*The rod-like portion of the myosin molecule may contain three parallel chains: there is controversy on this point and it is not settled.

Figure 1. *The sarcomere is delimited at either end by the very electron-dense Z band (Z). From the Z bands at either end of the unit, the thin filaments pass centrally to interdigitate with the thick filaments. The latter make up the A band (A); the I Band (I) is the portion of the sarcomere where the thin filaments exist alone. M = the system of cross linkages which holds the thick filaments in rigid array and marks the center of the contractile unit. (x 153,333).*

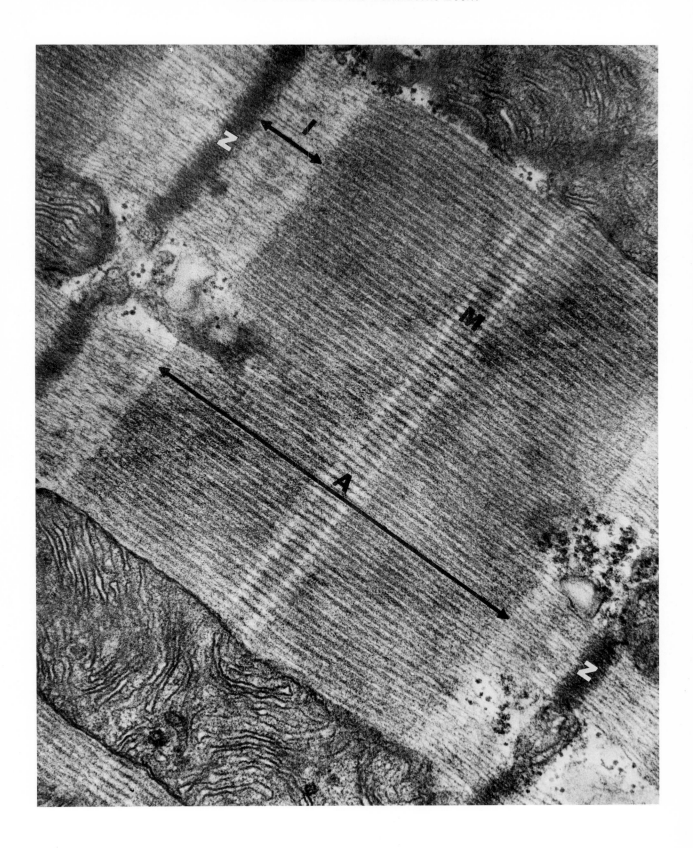

Figure 2. *This is a cross-section of the myofilaments and shows the hexagonal grouping of myosin around a central thick filament (1). Note that a sleeve of thin filaments in turn surrounds each thick filament, also in a hexagonal arrangement (2), and that each thin filament by virtue of its position can interact with three thick filaments simultaneously (3). (x 72,549).*

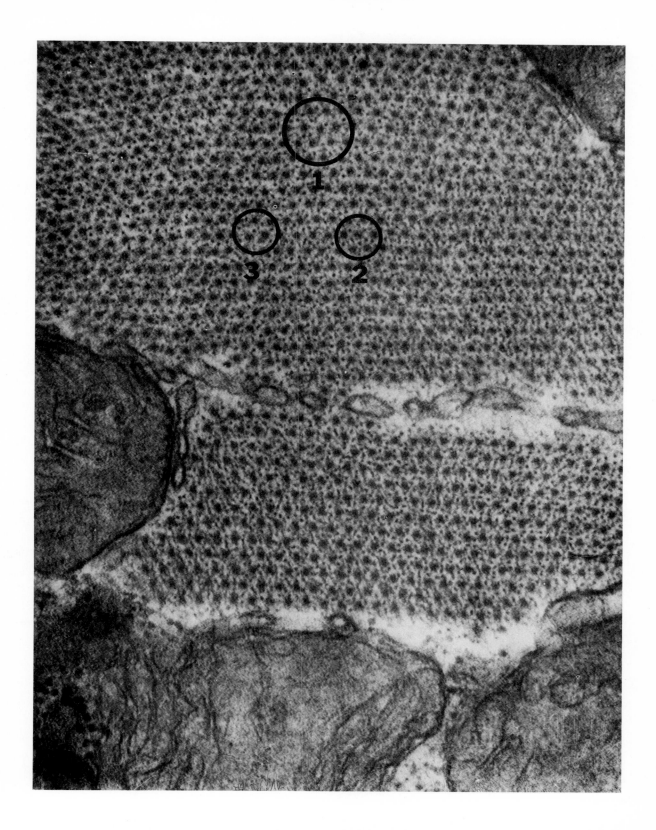

Figure 3. *This sketch of the sarcomere shows the thin filament as a double strand of beads, one wound about the other in a helical pattern. Note that the periodicity of the helix (each turn of which includes 6 molecules of globular (G) actin) is slightly less than that of the active site (AS) on the filament. The long, thin tropomyosin molecule (T) only one of which is represented on each thin filament (there are two, in actual fact) lies in the groove between the beaded strands of F-actin. Myosin molecules in an orderly array make up the thick filament, their globular bi-partite heads or cross bridges (CB) projecting from the molecule to lie in close proximity to the active sites on the thin filament. Note that their arrangement is reversed in the midline and that their bare, long stalks make up the body of the thick filament. They are held in rigid array by the system of cross linkages known collectively as the M-band (M).*

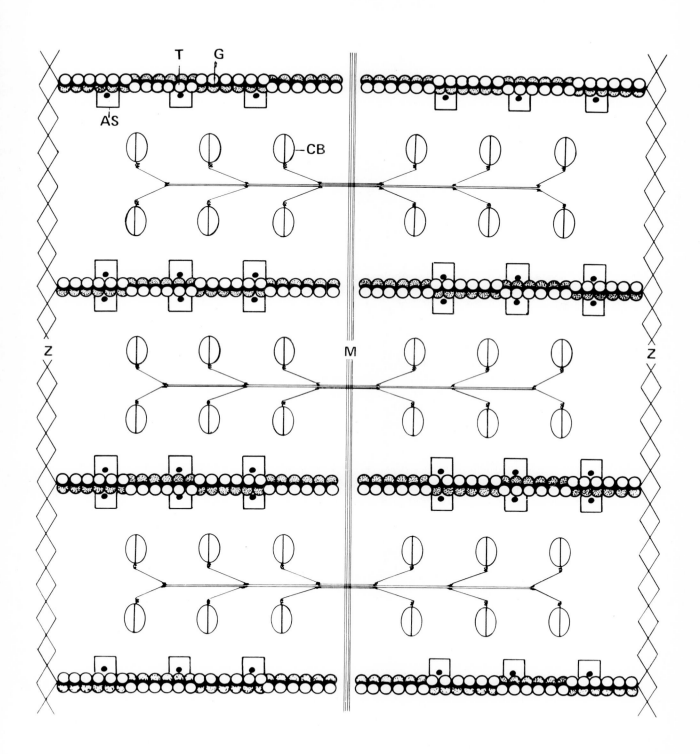

Figure 4. *This high power view of the Z band shows the Y-shaped insertion of the thin filament in the Z-substance (circle). Note that the Y figure is offset half a unit from the Y of the opposing thin filament. Each Y represents two of the four strands in which the thin filament terminates, each leg forming one of the four corners of a square when the configuration is viewed on end. The I-band filaments are in rigid parallel array for a short distance after their exit from the Z substance; then they pursue a more irregular course (see text). (x 93,333).*

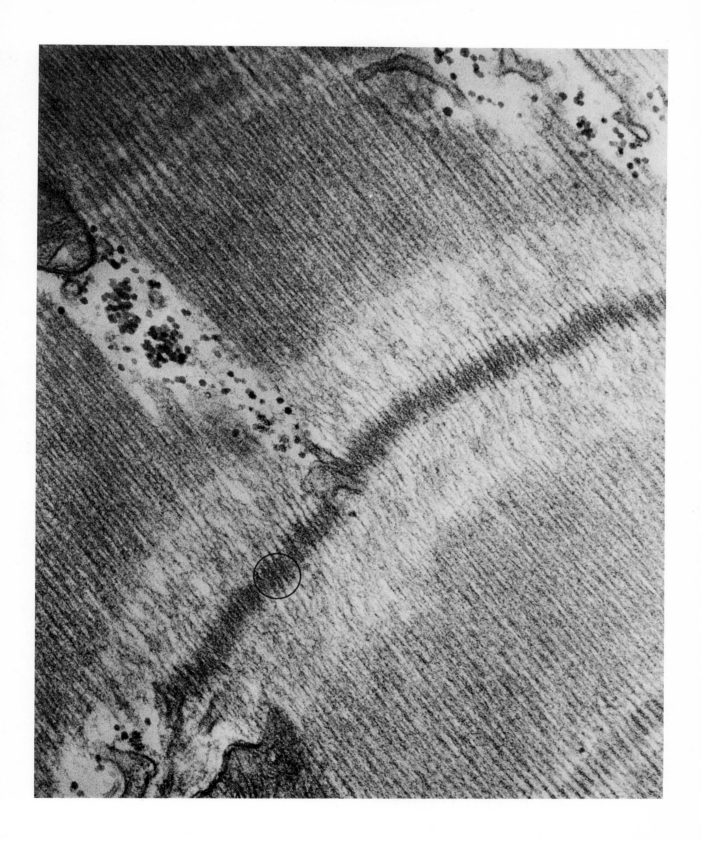

subunits. If, on the other hand, the myosin molecule is subjected to digestion with trypsin, it breaks into two fragments; one, called light meromyosin (LMM) has a molecular weight of 150,000 and is a straight rod, about 900 Å in length; the other, called heavy meromyosin (HMM), which consists of the globular head of the molecule attached to a short (400 Å) straight stalk, has a molecular weight of 350,000 (Figure 5) (12, 13). It is these two fragments of the myosin molecule we shall discuss in detail, (remembering that it is the heavy meromyosin portion of the molecule which contains the light chains obtained by treatment with urea).

Slayter and Lowey in 1967 suggested from observation of the HMM portion of the molecule in the electron microscope that HMM is, in fact, *bipartite* and consists of two helical stalks on each of which is mounted a globular head (14); whether or not there are two separate globular heads or a single, although bipartite, head that acts as a unit, is a point of confusion about the myosin molecule. Most investigators, however, postulate that there are two components to the globular portion of the myosin molecule, as we shall see later in our discussion of the shortening mechanism.

The HMM fragment of the myosin is the portion of the molecule that makes contact with the active sites on the thin filament during sarcomeric shortening. It is called a "cross bridge," therefore, since it crosses the gap between the two major sarcomeric components in the contractile event.

The myosin molecules are stacked together to form the thick filaments in the following way; the middle $0/15\mu - 0/2\mu$ of the thick filament is without cross-bridges, the so-called bare area of the filament. At this bare area, the clustering of the myosin molecules at the center of the stalk begins with myosins being stacked together, their stalks almost parallel to the long axis of the filament and their "cross bridge" portion extending from the surface of the unit (Figure 3). The myosin molecules in either half of the filament are arranged in opposite senses so that the two halves of the filament are mirror images of each other. This happens in the following way (15): from the central portion of the filament, myosin molecules are arranged in a repeating sequence or pattern in groups of six. They are stacked together so that, in any group of six sequentially arranged molecules, three pairs of two cross bridges, each one of a pair located opposite the other in the filament, wind around the circumference of the filament in a helical path. Each pair is 143Å distant from the previous pair; moreover, as they progress along the filament, each doublet rotates 120° further around the circumference of the filament than the previous pair. Hence, with three sets of cross bridges, the helix makes a complete turn; this is called a "6/2 helix" or a helix with "three-fold screw symmetry." The pitch of the helix so formed is 143 Å x 3 or 429 Å (15).

The finished thick filament is 1.5μ long and is composed of two halves, each one the mirror-image structurally of the other, and is covered on all sides by projections (Huxley estimates there may be as many as 200—250, per thick filament) which are the heavy meromyosin portions of the myosin molecules. Except for a central bare area of $0/15\mu - 0/2\mu$, these cross bridges are so arranged that they pursue an orderly helical path in pairs of two around the circumference of the filament (Figure 6). The LMM portions of the major molecule make up the thick, linear portion of the filament, and are bound to one another in a roughly parallel fashion along the entire length of the filament. The cross bridges extend as projections from the surface of the filament.

Hugh Huxley observed that in the transition from relaxation, when no cross bridges were in contact, to rigor, when vitually all myosin's cross bridges were engaged by the thin filaments, cross bridges were able to move both radially and circumferentially around the thick filament, with only their base fixed at 143 Å intervals (15). He postulated the existence of a flexible link between the LMM and HMM fragments which would allow this type of movement by the cross bridge around a fixed point at its base at the point of exit from the thick filament, and supported his contention by the observation that, as we have said, trypsin digestion divided the molecule in two at this point. He also postulated the existence of a second flexible link joining the globular head of the HMM fragment to its stalk, pointing out that the orientation of the globular head had to be correctly maintained so that, as the cross bridge moved either radially or circumferentially around the long axis of the thick filament, the orientation of the polar head would be such that its interaction with the active site on the thin filament was still possible (15, 16).

In summary then, the finished thick filament is more or less cylindrical (actually it has a rather triangular shape in cross-section, probably due to the way LMM is stacked together) whose structure, and hence whose polarity, from the point of view of molecular arrangement in each half of the unit, is reversed in the midline. Apart from a short (1/15—1/20 of the total length of the filament) middle portion which is smooth or "bare," the surface of the cylinder is made up of pairs of cross bridges (which are globular heads on short stalks) separated from each other by 180°, one each on opposite sides of the filament. The cross bridge pairs march in a helical sequence out to either ends of the filament from the central bare area, the pitch of the helix being completed with three sets of cross bridges, a total distance of 429 Å. The cross bridges, estimated to be about 200-250 in number per thick filament, move both radially and circumferentially in space, fixed only at their base portion. The body of the thick filament itself is composed of the light meromyosin portion of the myosin molecule.

If we examine the way thick and thin filaments are arranged in the sarcomere, it will become apparent why the arrangement of cross bridges all around the circumference of the myosin filament is necessary (Figure 6). The thick filaments themselves, when viewed in cross-section are arranged in a hexagonal pattern around a central myosin unit. Six thick filaments are grouped in turn, around each myosin. Each thick filament reacts with six thin filaments, then; the latter enclose the myosin in a virtual sleeve. Conversely, the position of the thin filament is such that each one can interact with three myosin filaments simultaneously during the contractile event (Figure 2).

Huxley points out the necessity for the cross bridges to be mobile and still retain the correct orientation of their polarized globular heads with respect to the active sites on the thin filament: the distance between filaments is not constant, but varies with sarcomeric length (or to put it another way, with degree of muscle stretch) (15, 16). The thin filaments move closer to the thick filament as the sarcomere lengthens; they are further apart when the sarcomere shortens.* Cross

---

*This is a useful phenomenon, if one considers that there are opposing electrostatic forces operating between filaments which serve to maintain a low coefficient of friction between the strands as they move past one another. As the degree of overlap between thick and thin filaments becomes less with sarcomeric lengthening or stretch, they move closer together, and the electrostatic forces between the remaining portions become stronger, maintaining the friction coefficient at a constant low level.)

Figure 5. This is a sketch of the myosin molecule, showing the two helical chains that form the stalk of the molecule and which extend upward to end in the bi-partite globular head portion of the molecule. The two "hinged" areas of the molecule, which are susceptible to trypsin digestion, are indicated. The proposed area of the "light chain" subunits of the molecule, which result from urea treatment, and in which the ATPase property of the molecule resides, are indicated by blacked-in areas. HMM_1 = heavy meromyosin subfragment one. HMM_2 = heavy meromyosin subfragment two. LMM = light meromyosin subfragment. LC = light chain. The insert indicates the manner in which the myosin molecule will be represented in all future sketches.

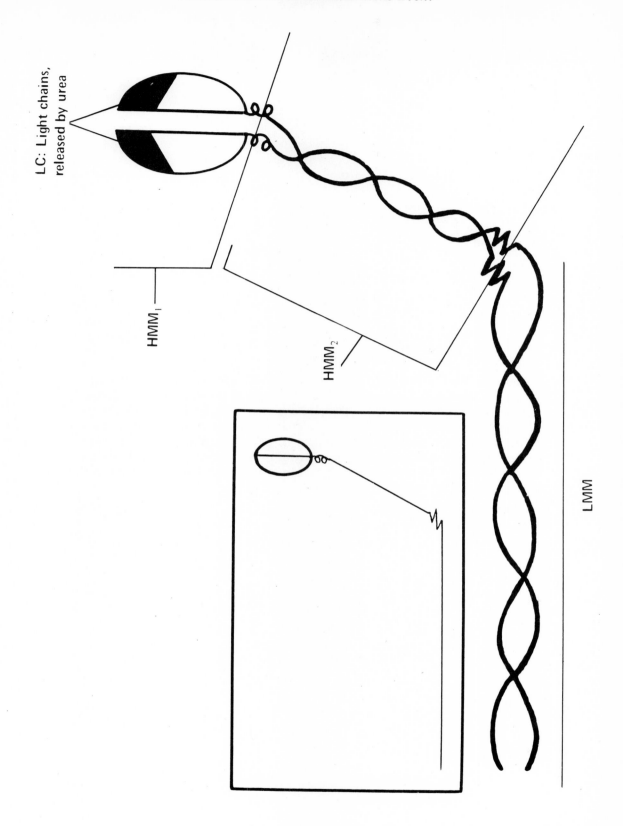

LC: Light chains, released by urea

HMM₁

HMM₂

LMM

Figure 6. *This is a sketch of a small portion of a hexagonal array of myosin filaments viewed so that the helical arrangement of cross bridges on each of the thick filaments is seen. The multiplicity of cross bridges, and their availability for interaction with active sites on a multiplicity of thin filaments are apparent. (For simplicity, no thin filaments have been included in this diagram, but each myosin filament is surrounded by six thin filaments in the sarcomere). CB = cross bridge. MF = myosin filament.)*

Portion of myosin (thick) filament (MF)

Cross bridge on
thick filament (CB)

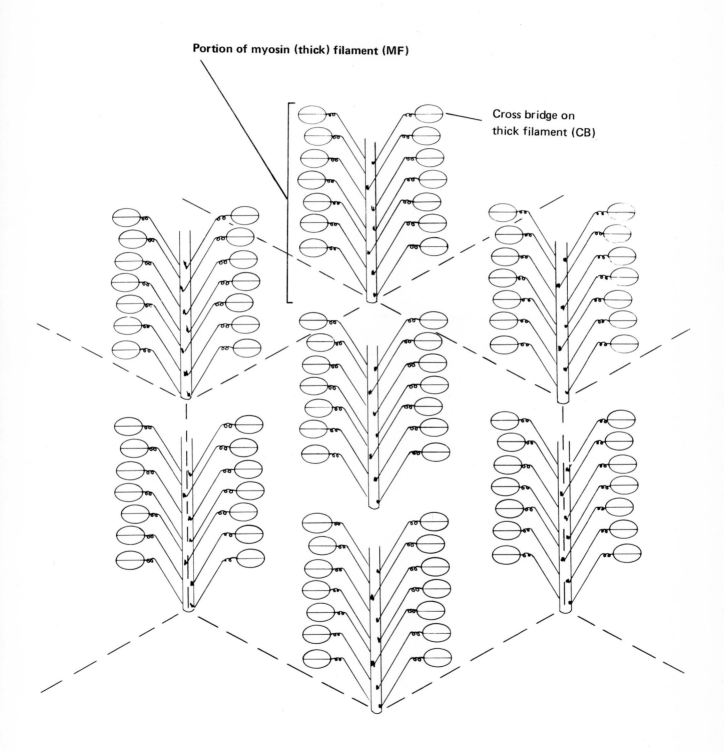

Figure 7. *This is a sketch of the sliding filament mechanism of muscular contraction as envisaged by Hugh Huxley. In this model, 1. the globular head (CB) of the myosin molecule makes no contact with the active site (AS) on the thin filament until calcium is added to the system. 2. Calcium changes the troponin molecule configuration so that interaction is possible between the two filaments and cross bridge-active site contact is made. 3. The two portions of the myosin ATPase then change their alignment with respect to one another; in so doing, they move the active site and with it the entire thin filament a short distance toward the center of the sarcomere. 4. The original configuration of the myosin head is then re-established with the rupture of the active site-cross bridge link, and the cross bridge is ready for interaction with a new active site on a thin filament. ATP is split at some point in this sequence; exactly where, however, we do not know.*

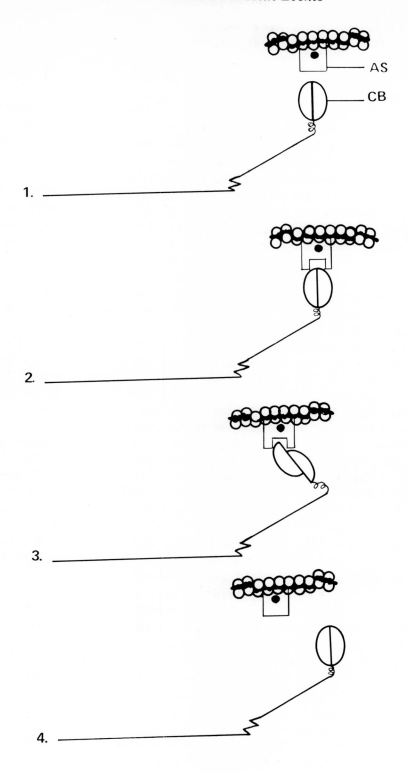

AS

CB

1.

2.

3.

4.

Mechanism of sliding filament hypothesis (Huxley)

bridges must be able to move their long axis more parallel to that of the thin filament when inter-filament distance is less at long sarcomere lengths, or on the other hand, to position themselves on their long axis more perpendicular to that of the body of the thick filament as interfilamentous distances increase at short sarcomere lengths.

While the exact mechanism of filament interaction to produce sarcomeric shortening is really not known, certain fundamental facts are clear; neither the position or length of thick filaments is changed in the contractile event; the A band remains the same length and occupies the same central position in the sarcomere. What does happen is that the thin filaments are moved centrally from either end of the sarcomere, sliding past the stationary thick filaments and causing the Z- to -Z distance to shorten. This movement is occasioned by the interaction that occurs between the active site on the thin filament and the globular head on the myosin cross bridge; links between the thin and thick filaments are sequentially made and broken. With each successive reaction, the thin filament moves a certain distance, perhaps, Huxley calculates, as little as 8 Å. ATP is split with each contact between the cross bridge and the active site, although we do not know exactly at what moment in the sequence this occurs, or how the energy so released is utilized.

There is more than one theory of how the thin filaments actually are made to slide past the thick in the contractile event. One of the most attractive, simplest, and best known is that of Huxley (15, 16), who suggests that a simple rearrangement of the two portions of the globular head of the myosin fragment will occasion sliding of the actin filament in the following way (Figure 7):

The two portions of the globular head of the cross bridge make contact with the active site on the thin filament. They then undergo a simple repositioning with respect to one another that causes an angulation of the head towards the center of the sarcomere. This moves the active site (still attached to the now angulated head of the myosin molecule and with it the entire thin filament) toward the sarcomere's center. The cross bridge—active site link is then broken, the two portions of the globular head resume their original orientation and the angulation of the head is lost. The now restored and erect head is ready to react with another active site on a thin filament. This sequential making and breaking of cross bridges is what moves the thin filaments from either end of the contractile unit toward the sarcomeric center.

Huxley points out that the reversal of polarity in the mid-portion of the thick filaments (and hence the entire A band) is essential to the proper direction of movement of the thin filament: each group of sarcomeric thin filaments must move in opposite directions, i.e.: each group moves from the Z band at the end of the sarcomere, toward each other; if both groups of thin filaments moved in the same direction, the Z to Z distance would not shorten and no contraction would occur. For the same reason, the I band filaments at either end of the sarcomere must have opposite polarities.

It is probable that a single molecule of ATP is split by one cross bridge for each cycle of its action—this is a very efficient system, because the amount of energy consumed is exactly equal to and indeed, determined by, the amount of work done in the myofiber.

Interaction between sarcomeric components cannot occur without the calcium ion: calcium changes the configuration of the tropomyosin—troponin complex blocking the active sites on the thin filament, allowing them to interact with myosin's cross bridges (17). Both the amount of calcium presented to the sarcomere and the duration of time it is left at the level of the myofilaments will determine the total number of cross bridge—active site combinations that occur and hence the amount of movement of the thin filaments along myosin. As we see, then, calcium is not only the link in the cell between excitation and contraction, but it determines the degree of sarcomeric shortening and hence how much systolic force is generated by the cell. The amount of calcium at the releasing site (which is probably the perimembrane, or external lamina of the cell, as we have discussed in Chapter Two) which enters the level of the myofilaments as a consequence of excitation, directly determines how rapidly force is developed by the cell (the rate of force development is referred to as dP/dt). To say it another way, the intensity of the active state in the cell, is a function of the amount of calcium at any given instant at the level of the myofilaments. Calcium entry into the cell continues as long as the action potential continues; the duration of time during which calcium continues to enter the cell determines the duration of the active state (or the time to peak tension, TPT). It follows that if one is to increase contraction one must do so by either delivering more calcium to the system no matter what kind of inotropic intervention is chosen, or by letting it remain for a longer time at the level of the sarcomere.

Specific References

1. Leeuwenhoek, A. van.: *The Collected Letters of Antoni van Leeuwenhoek.* Ed. by a Committee of Dutch Scientists. Zeitlinger, Swets & Amsterdam, 1939.
2. Huxley, H. E.: Electron Microscope Studies on the Structure of Natural and Synthetic Protein Filaments from Striated Muscle. *J. Mol. Biol.,* 7:281, 1963.
3. Sakabibara, I. and Yagi, K.: Molecular Weight of G—Actin Obtained by the Light Scattering Method. *Biochem. Biophys. Act.,* **207**:178, 1970.
4. Hanson, J. and Lowy, J.: The Structure of F-Actin Filaments Isolated From Muscle. *J. Mol. Biol.,* 6:46, 1963.
5. Maruyama, K.: Effect of β-Actinin on the Particle Length of F-Actin. *Biochem. Biophys. Acta,* **126**:389, 1966.
6. Kawaura, M. and Maruyama, K.: Electron Microscopic Particle Length of F—Actin Polymerized in Vitro. *J. Bio. Chem.,* 67:437, 1970.
7. Masaki, T., Endo, M., and Ebashi, S.: Localization of 6 S Component of α-Actinin at Z Band. *J. Biochem.,* 62:630, 1967.
8. Franzini-Armstrong, C.: Details of the I Band Structure as Revealed by the Localization of Ferritin. *Tissue & Cell,* 2:327, 1970.
9. Ohtsuki, I., Masaki, T., Nonamura, Y., and Ebashi, S.: Periodic Distribution of Troponin along the Thin Filament. *J. Biochem.,* 61:817, 1967.
10. Greaser, M. L. and Gergely, J.: Reconstitution of Troponin Activity from Three Protein Components. *J. Biol. Chem.,* 246:4226, 1971.
11. Tsao, T. C.: Fragmentation of the Myosin Molecule. *Biochem. Biophys. Acta,* 11:368, 1953.
12. Gergley, J.: Studies on Myosin-adenosinetriphosphatase. *J. Biol. Chem.,* **200**:543, 1953.
13. Szent—Gyorgyi, A. G.: Meromyosins, the Subunits of Myosin. *Arch. Biochem. Biophys.,* 42:305, 1953.
14. Slayter, H. S. and Lowey, S.: Substructure of the Myosin Molecule as Visualized by Electron Microscopy. *Proc. Nat. Acad. Sci.,* 58:1611, 1967.

15. Huxley, H. E. and Brown, W.: The Low-angle X-Ray Diagram of Vertebrate Striated Muscle and Its Behaviour During Contraction and Rigor. *J. Mol. Biol.*, **30**:383, 1967.
16. Huxley, H. E.: The Mechanism of Muscular Contraction. *Science*, **164**:1356, 1969.
17. Ebashi, S., Ebashi, F., and Kodama, A.: Troponin as the Ca++ Receptive Protein in the Contractile System. *J. Biochem.*, **62**:137, 1967.

General References

Hodge, A. J.: Fibrous Proteins of Muscle. *Rev. Mod. Physics.*, **31**:45, 1959.

Katz, A. M.: Contractile Proteins of the Heart. *Physiol. Rev.* **50**:63 1970.

Katz, A. M.: Contractile Proteins in Normal and Failing Myocardium. *Hos. Prac.* 7:57, 1972.

Dreizen, P. and Gershman, T. C.: Molecular Basis of Muscular Contraction, Myosin. *Trans. of N. Y. Acad. Sci.*, **32**:170, 1970.

CHAPTER IV

The Mitochondrion

Mitochondria, or sarcosomes, are the energy-producing units of the myofiber. They are very abundant in cardiac muscle and lie packed in rows between myofibrils in close proximity to the sarcomeric units, to which they supply energy for the contractile event (Figure 1). The mitochondrion is an interesting entity: without it, the cell cannot respire; there is no equipment for aerobic metabolism in the sarcoplasm.

Mitochondria are self sufficient in many respects; unlike the other components of the cell, they are not entirely produced and maintained under the direction and control of nuclear DNA. They contain their own DNA and, what is more, it is not the double helix of nuclear DNA, but is a circular filament like that of bacteria or viruses (1). Unlike nuclear DNA, moreover, it is often membrane associated. The mitochondrion reproduces by fission and distributes genetic material to the two-daughter units (Figures 2, 3, 4).

The fact that the mitochondrion possesses its own genetic information makes it relatively independent of the rest of the cell; mitochondria synthesize their own proteins and phospholipids. These make up their elaborate inner membrane system, which has an enormous surface area arranged in complex involutions and foldings called cristae. It is upon these cristae that the energy produced when a substrate is metabolized is trapped for use by the cell via the manufacture of adenosine triphosphate (ATP). ATP thus produced is exported to the exterior of the mitochondrion, its terminal phosphate bond hydrolyzed and the resultant energy utilized for cell work.

The genetic independence of the mitochondrion and its ability to respire for the cell which otherwise is unable to metabolize aerobically, have prompted the speculation that the mitochondrion is an inclusion body within the cell, self-maintaining and self-replicating, existing in a kind of optimal symbiosis with its host (2).

Myocardial Metabolism and the Mitochondrion:

General Characteristics of Myocardial Metabolism

The heart works rhythmically and without stopping. Its work performance is relatively constant, in contrast to skeletal muscle, where activity comes in spurts and there can be rest periods during which energy stores are replenished without danger to life. The myocardium must metabolize at a rate that closely parallels the amount of work done, and it must do so with relatively high efficiency. This necessity for a constant level of high energy compounds makes certain features of cardiac metabolism unique: for example, the heart's concentration of creatinine phosphate (CP) is low: creatinine phosphate's function is to replenish ATP in the cell. It does this by transferring a high energy phosphate bond from its own molecule to that of adenosine diphosphate. Creatinine phosphate is a useful compound for skeletal muscle; there is leisure to replace ATP slowly after bursts of activity. But cardiac muscle must maintain constantly high levels of ATP and has less use for the CP-ATP phosphate transfer.

While the heart can utilize glucose anaerobically to maintain life, it becomes evident, for reasons we shall discuss in detail, that the myocardium must, in general, metabolize foodstuffs aerobically in order to be effective; aerobic metabolism is vastly more efficient than anaerobic metabolism. This explains the high arterio-venous oxygen difference across the coronary circulation in comparison to the rest of the systemic circulation. The heart is also protected by the versatility with which it can extract substrates from the blood: it must be able to function in starvation states and, while it preferentially selects glucose as a substrate in the fed or replenished organism, it can use fatty acids for as much as 70% of its total substrate in the starved or fasting situation. Another protection for the myocardium is its ability to store glycogen; glycogen granules are universally present and abundant in the myofibers, especially in those with specialized conducting or pacing tasks to perform. This glycogen provides a buffer for the cell in a nutrient-deprived state.

Cardiac Metabolism and the Citric Acid Cycle

To be effective, the metabolism of food stuff by the cell should be efficient and proceed virtually isothermically. The energy released should not be in the form of heat to any significant extent; such a consequence of substrate processing would threaten the constant temperature of the cell—a temperature which must be maintained within very narrow limits if cellular processes are to proceed optimally. The energy produced by metabolic processes should be maximally conserved, moreover, and converted into a form which can be stored for use at another, later time, until it is needed for the performance of cellular work. It is for these reasons that substrates such as glycogen, glucose and fats are broken down by the cell in multiple stages: with successive transformation of the foodstuff, energy is released in small quantities and funneled piecemeal, as it were, via the co-enzymes of the electron transport chain into the manufacture of ATP, a compound with a terminal high-energy phosphate bond. ATP is stored by the cell until energy is needed for work, at which time, the phosphate bond is ruptured and the energy released for utilization.

The respiring mitochondrion breaks down food stuff, or substrate, by a sequence of oxidations (the loss of electrons and with them H+ ions or protons; oxidation, therefore is also called dehydrogenation), and eventually transforms these into CO2 and H_2O. The electrons so released are transferred one at a time, in an orderly sequence along a series of compounds called co-enzymes. Co-enzymes have varying affinities for electrons. The electrons, therefore, flow in a predictable sequence along this series of compounds, the so called "electron-transport chain," moving from the co-enzyme with the lowest affinity for electrons (or "redox potential," as it is called) to that with the highest, eventually combining with oxygen. In the process of repetitive transfer of electrons from one co-enzyme to the next, energy is released and utilized for the manufacture of ATP. Oxidation of foodstuff or substrate, then, is closely coupled to the production of ATP: this whole process is called oxidative phosphorylation. When the ratio of molecules of O_2 consumed to the molecules of phosphate utilized for the manufacture of ATP is about 1:3, the cell's metabolism is characterized as "tightly coupled"; if substrate oxidation does not result in the phosphorylation of ADP, the cell is "uncoupled."

The sequence of reactions by which all foodstuffs are eventually oxidized and by which the electrons so released are provided to the transport system, is called the citric acid cycle (CAC), (Table 1). In this cycle of reactions, pyruvic acid, which is the compound formed in the cell cytoplasm by the decarboxylation and dehydrogenation of glucose, is transported into the mitochondrion, where it enters a reaction sequence which begins with its transformation into acetyl coenzyme A (acetyl CoA); acetyl CoA is a key compound in metabolism in that it is the end product not only of the cytoplasmic processing glucose (and hence of carbohydrate) but also the compound into which fatty acids are eventually metabolized. This happens when the carbon chain of the fatty acid is broken into two-carbon fragments by a process of repetitive β-decarboxylation and attachment of the double carbon piece to co-enzyme A to form acetyl CoA. Proteins, broken down into their component amino acids, also enter the CAC cycle by deamination and a transfer of their NH_2 group, with the eventual production of either pyruvate or acetyl CoA.

Acetyl CoA is condensed with the four-carbon containing molecule of oxaloacetic acid to form citric acid. This begins the tri-carboxylic acid or citric acid cycle. A series of reactions, which includes hydrolysis, oxidative decarboxylations, hydration and finally oxidation, ends with the regeneration of oxaloacetic acid. This reaction sequence, called a "cycle" because it is self regenerative, continues as long as acetyl CoA is available, (Table 1) and is, obviously, the major final common oxygen-utilizing pathway of carbohydrate, fat and protein breakdown in the cell.

For each turn of the citric acid cycle, one acetyl CoA molecule is consumed and two molecules of CO_2 are evolved. Three of the CAC reactions produce electron transfer to the most common co-enzyme or member of the electron transport chain: diphosphopyridinenucleotide (DPN+, also called NAD+). The oxidation of DPNH via the electron transport chain produces most of the energy available from respiration. (Other important co-enzymes making up the electron-transport chain are flavinmononucleotide (FMN) or flavineadeninedinucleotide (FAD) which are tightly bound to their dehydrogenases and are called flavoproteins; co-enzyme Q or ubiquinone, the cyctochromes b, c, a and a_3 and finally, cytochrome oxidase.)

ATP is formed at three steps along the electron transport chain, generating a total of 12 moles of ATP for each molecule of acetyl CoA going through the citric acid cycle. One mole of glucose, then, will be metabolized with the production of 24 moles of ATP as a consequence of the metabolism of pyruvate by the citric acid cycle, (1 glucose = 2 acetyl CoA = 24 ATP molecules via each revolution of the cycle.)

There are two other points at which ATP is produced during the processing of glucose: When pyruvate enters the mitochondrion and is changed into acetyl CoA, two molecules of DPNH are produced: the oxidation of these provides 6 moles of

TABLE 1.

THE PRODUCTION OF 38 MOLES OF ATP FROM ONE MOLECULE OF GLUCOSE ANAEROBICALLY IN THE CYTOPLASM AND AEROBICALLY IN THE MITOCHONDRION.

ANAEROBIC METABOLISM: NET PRODUCTION OF 2 MOLES OF ATP FOR EACH MOLE OF GLUCOSE METABOLISED.

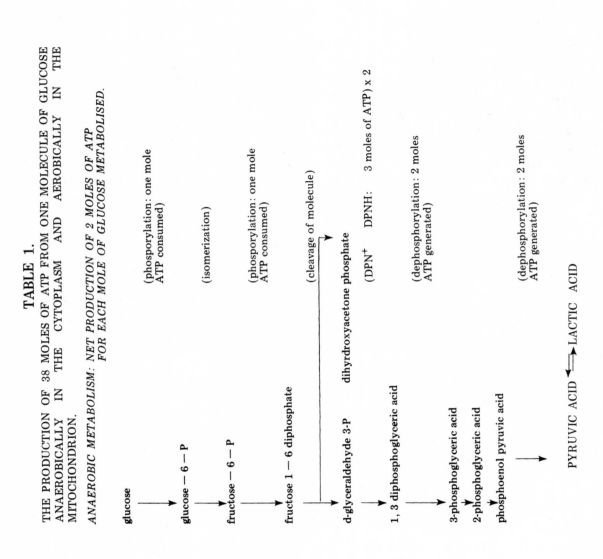

glucose

glucose — 6 — P   (phosporylation: one mole ATP consumed)

fructose — 6 — P   (isomerization)

fructose 1 — 6 diphosphate   (phosporylation: one mole ATP consumed)

d-glyceraldehyde 3-P   dihydroxyacetone phosphate   (cleavage of molecule)

1, 3 diphosphoglyceric acid   (DPN^+ DPNH: 3 moles of ATP) x 2

3-phosphoglyceric acid   (dephosphorylation: 2 moles ATP generated)

2-phosphoglyceric acid

phosphoenol pyruvic acid   (dephosphorylation: 2 moles ATP generated)

PYRUVIC ACID ⇌ LACTIC ACID

AEROBIC METABOLISM (INTRAMITOCHONDRIAL): NET PRODUCTION OF 36 MOLES OF ATP GENERATED FOR EACH MOLE OF GLUCOSE METABOLIZED.

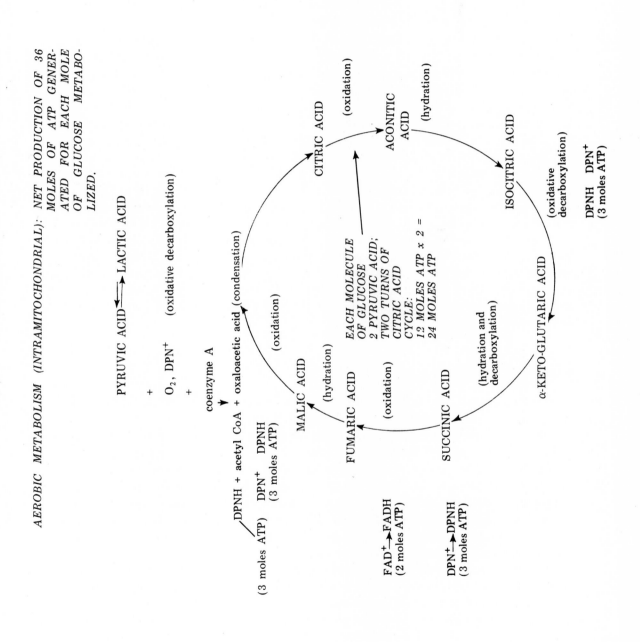

ATP per glucose equivalent: (DPNH $\rightarrow$ DPN$^+$ + H$^+$ + 3ATP). Two moles of DPNH are also produced in the cytoplasm during the processing of glucose (the production of 1-3 diphosphoglyceric acid from d - glyceraldehyde 3-PO$_4$); another 6 moles of ATP are generated when this DPNH is re-oxidized.

The total ATP produced by the aerobic metabolism of glucose is 2 + 6 + 6 + 24 or 38 moles of ATP. Now, the oxidation of glucose to CO_2 + H_2O produces 686,000 calories. Each mole of (ADP + P) $\rightarrow$ ATP formed requires 8,000 calories; it therefore follows that (38 x 8,000 =) 304,000 calories of the 686,000 calories available are conserved: this is an efficiency of 45%.

If pyruvate is not aerobically metabolized, the cytoplasm must metabolize it and extrude it from the cell without oxygen consumption: this is done with the regeneration of DPN+ and the reduction of pyruvate to lactate. No net energy is harnessed in this operation—the reduction of DPN$^+$ to DPNH consumes energy (3 moles of ATP) in the cell. This is balanced by the regeneration of DPN$^+$, which produces 3 moles of ATP. The only ATP produced in the anaerobic metabolism of glucose is a net of 2 moles for each mole of glucose consumed: this conserves 16,000 calories of the 56,000 calories produced in the transformation of glucose to lactate, an efficiency of 30%. Further, if one considers that the metabolism of glucose to lactate releases only 56,000 of the potential 686,000 calories available if it is totally degraded to CO_2 and H_2O; anaerobic use of glucose releases only 8.5% or less than 10% of the total potential energy of the foodstuff. In contrast, aerobic metabolism releases all the calories available, although only about half of these can be conserved. The anaerobic process has 5% of the efficiency of the aerobic process for the cell. It becomes clear, then, that at least in the case of glucose utilization, the cell is infinitely better off respiring than it is anaerobically metabolizing. Hence, the usefulness to the myofiber of the mitochondrion is self-evident.

Mitochondrial Morphology

Morphologically, the mitochondrion of the cardiac cell is an elliptical organelle approximately 0/5μ wide and 1— 3μ long. It has an elaborately folded inner membrane which doubles back and forth across the entire thickness of the sarcosome in closely packed folds called "cristae." (Figure 5) The long axes of these cristae, in general, are perpendicular to the long axis of the mitochondrion, but they may be arranged in concentric whorls inside the unit, or lie parallel to the long axis of the sarcosome. They may even be almost randomly arranged, frequently changing direction inside the mitochondrion. The number of cristae is proportional to the rate at which the sarcosomes respire and produce energy; they are therefore very abundant in cardiac tissue.

Enclosing the entire inner membrane system is a protective envelope or outer sheath. This is synthesized under the control of nuclear DNA (1) and is morphologically identical with all the other smooth membrane systems of the cell, such as that of the sarcoplasmic reticular network. The outer membrane is capable of active transport and has enzymatic properties (3).

The inter-membranous space, and the intra-cristal spaces are filled with an amorphous phase which contains, among other things, soluble enzymes, electrolytes and even under some circumstances electron dense salts and crystalline material. DNA filaments and mitochondrial ribosomes are also present in the intra-cristal spaces. The inner membrane system is entirely made up of repeating units. These are tripartite and consist of a basepiece, a stalk and a globular head; the latter is called an "elementary body." (Figure 5).

The basepieces are lipoprotein units lined up side to side and which, if isolated from their head and stalk portion will re-unite to form a continuous membranous layer. The chemical composition of the basepiece is 30% phospholipid by weight and has a 1:1 ratio of enzymatic to structural protein (4).

Contained in the intracristal space are the soluble enzymes of the citric acid cycle and possibly the coenzymes Q (ubiquinone) and cytochrome C. The basepiece of the stalk has other of the citric acid cycle dehydrogenases and the coenzymes necessary for electron transport and ATP synthesis. Some of the enzymes of metabolism are present in the outer membrane and inter-membranous space; specifically those which are involved in the processing of the fatty acid ester of acetyl CoA which is manufactured in the extra-mitochondrial space and actively transported into the sarcosome for oxidation.

Energy Utilization in the Mitochondrion

How the energy released by the electron transport chain is actually utilized to form ATP is a matter of some controversy at this present time: there are several theories—one of which postulates the formation of a "high-energy intermediate" compound which combines with inorganic phosphate, eventually transferring it to ADP to manufacture ATP (5). No such compound or compounds have been isolated, however, and this theory cannot be substantiated at the present time.

The idea which is currently most popular is that actual high-energy configurational changes in the cristal membrane are utilized in the formation of ATP. This is the so-called configurational hypothesis, and is given considerable weight by the observation of many investigators that there are indeed configurational changes in the mitochondrion, sometimes very profound, that can be correlated with the state of respiration in the sarcosome (6, 7, 8). For example, depending on whether substrate, ADP, the electron transport chain or oxygen is the limiting factor in oxidative phosphorylation, various configurations can be produced in mitochondria in vitro or, alternately, correlated with their in vivo appearance in the cell.

Ion Transport by Mitochondria

Morphologic changes in the arrangement of the inner membrane system and even the over all shape of mitochondria occur as a consequence of their ability to transport ions—such changes do not seem to be purely the result of osmotically induced water shifts in and/or out of the sarcosome, moreover, but may represent, at least in part, true conformational changes in the cristal membrane itself. The ability of the mitochondrion to actively transport both anions and cations with the consumption of ATP or directly via the activity of the electron transport chain is probably an important regulatory factor in the control and maintenance of sarcoplasmic ionic composition. Some investigators believe that the ability of the mitochondrion to concentrate calcium ion or, alternately, release it, may play a role in sarcomeric relaxation and/or conceivably, in the regulation of systolic force in the cell (9), but these are by no means proven functions of the sarcosome. If it does indeed contribute, to systolic force generation by the myofiber, via control of the ionic milieu at the level of the myofiber, the quantitation of such a contribution would be very difficult.

Figure 1. *This electron micrograph shows portions of three cells, two joined by an intercalated disc (arrows). The relative size of the mitochondrion (M) and its position between sarcomeric units can be seen here. Note that at some sites they occur singly, while at others they exist in small pools. They vary markedly in size and shape; such variations are quite normal in the cardiac cell. (x 24,000).*

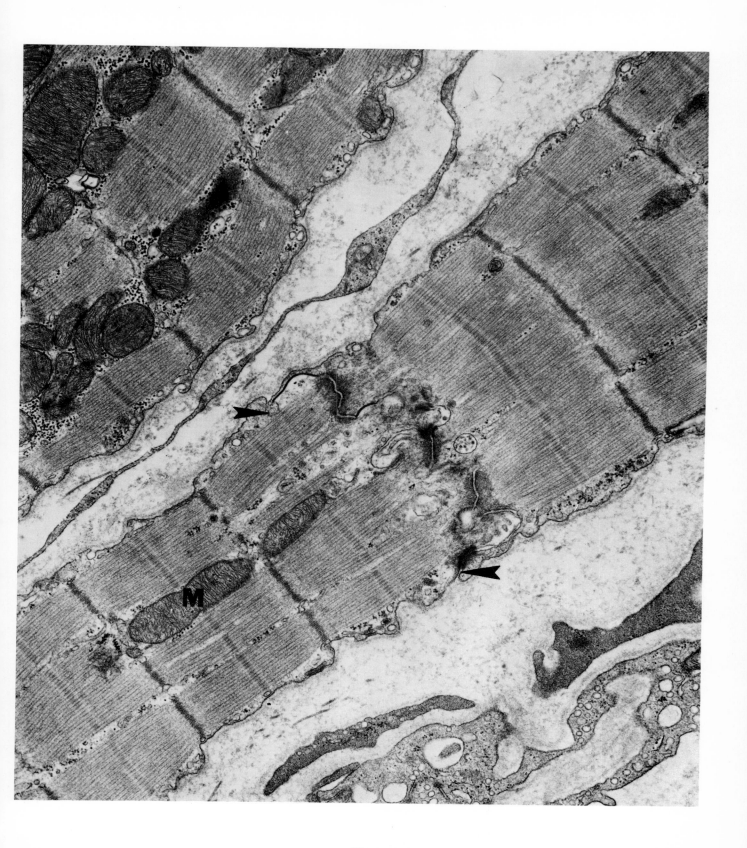

Figure 2. *These are young, simply constructed mitochondria (M) in a portion of a two day old rat ventricular cell grown in tissue culture. Note that they have relatively few cristae, which are arranged in an uncomplicated, widely spaced array. N = nucleus. (x 64,578).*

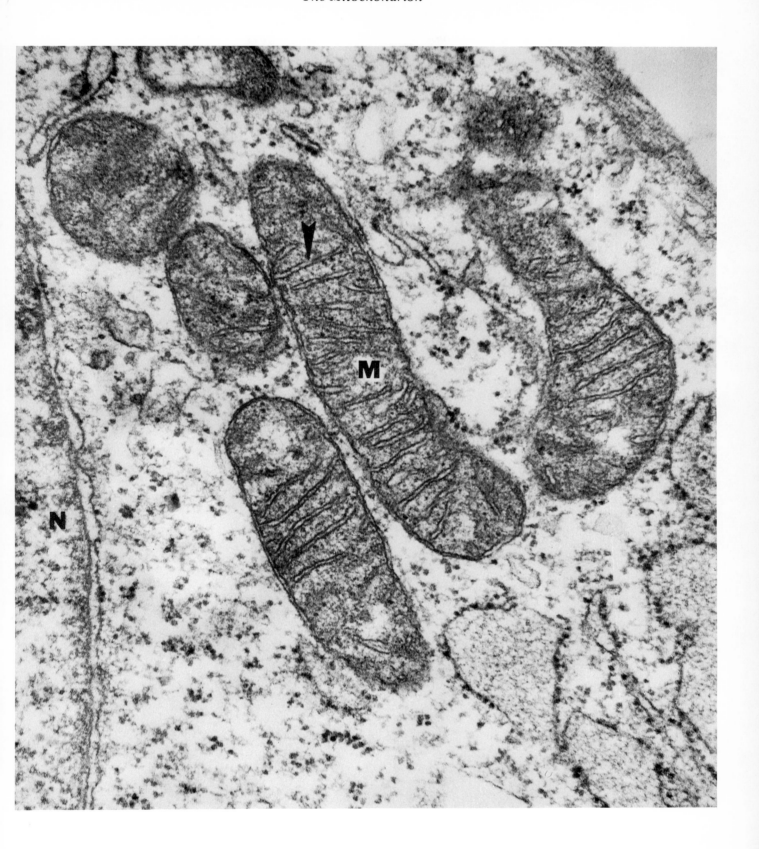

Figure 3. *This is a giant mitochondrion which has probably achieved maximal size in the same type of cell as is illustrated in Figure 2 (2 day old rat ventricular cell grown in tissue culture). Note the much more elaborate cristal arrangement and their close packing in the sarcosome. M = mitochondrion; N = nucleus. (Arrow points to a crista). (x 38,000).*

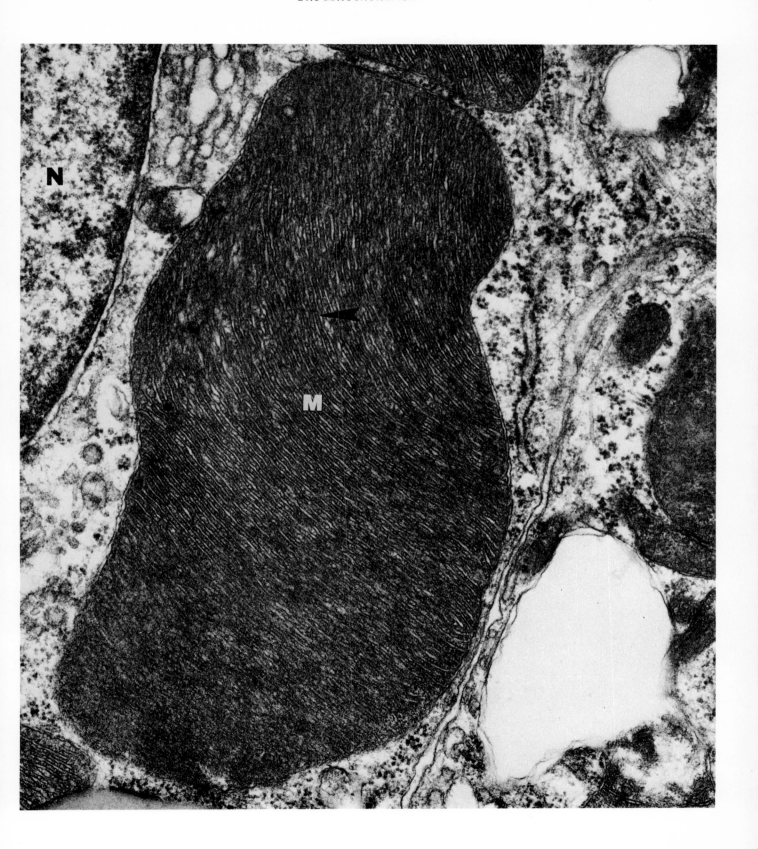

Figure 4. *This is an almost-divided mitochondrion, splitting to form two daughter units. Arrows mark the only remaining point of contact between them in this plane of the section. Again, the cell in which the sarcosomes lie is a 2-day old rat ventricular cell grown in tissue culture. (x 47,100).*

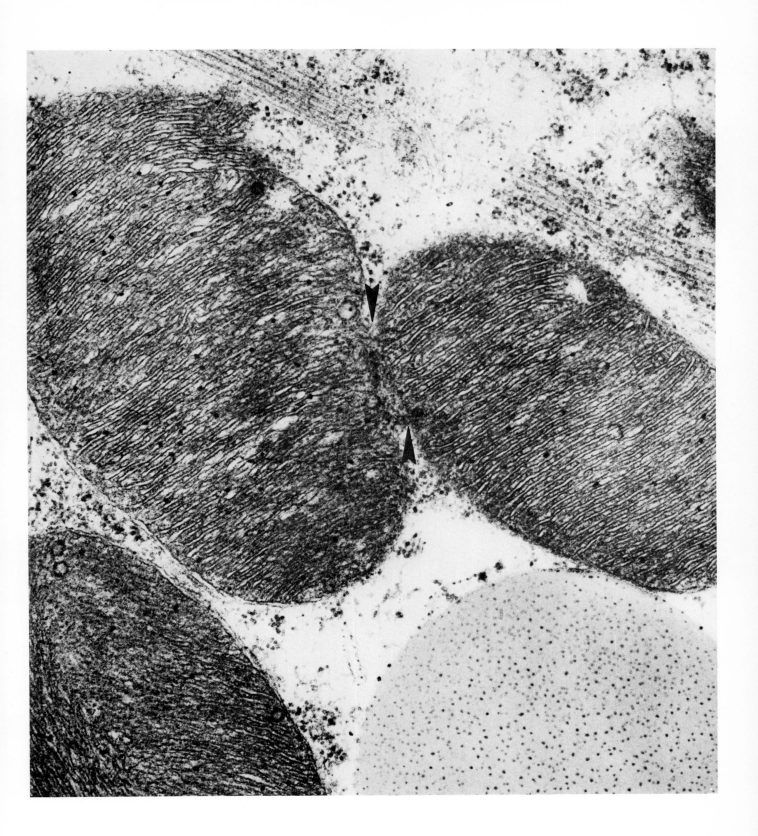

Figure 5. This sketch of the mitochondrion shows the difference between the outer membrane and the inner membrane system. The inner membrane is complexly folded within the space enclosed by the outer membrane to form cristae. The cristal membrane is composed of repeating tripartite units; these consist of base, stalk, and round headpiece (see text). We have not attempted to illustrate the molecular structure of the outer membrane in this diagram, but it is probably similar to that of other membrane systems in the cell such as smooth endoplasmic reticulum or the sarcolemma (see Chapter II).

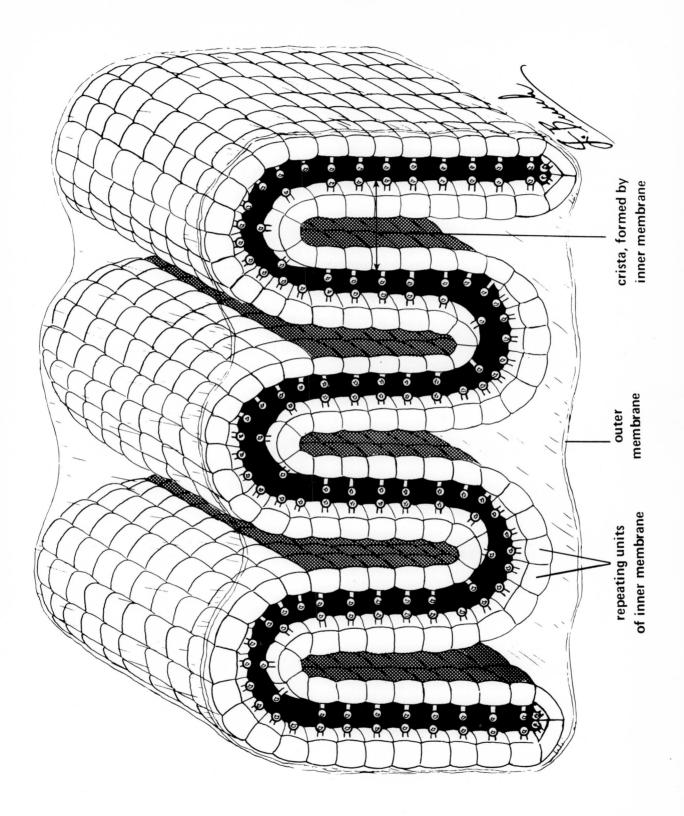

crista, formed by
inner membrane

outer
membrane

repeating units
of inner membrane

Specific References

1. Nass, M. M. K.: Mitochondrial DNA: Advances, Problems, and Goals. *Science*, **165**:25, 1969.
2. Thomas, L.: Notes of a Biology-Watcher: Organelles as Organisms. *N.E.J. Med.*, **287**:294, 1972.
3. Green, D. E., Allmann, R. A., and Tan, N. C.: Enzyme Localization in the Inner and Outer Mitochondrial Membranes. *Biochem. Biophys. Res. Comm.* **31**:368, 1968.
4. Green, D. E. and MacLennan, D. H.: Structure and Function of the Mitochondrial Membrane. *Bio. Science*, **19**:213, 1969.
5. Slater, E. C. and Holton, E. A.: Oxidative Phosphorylation Coupled with Oxidation of α-Keto Glutarate by Heart Muscle Sarcosomes. I. Kinetics of Oxidative Phosporylation Reaction and Adeninenucleotide Specificity. *Biochem. J.*, **55**:530, 1953.
6. Lehninger, A. L.: in *Horizons in Biochemistry*. Albert Szent-Györgyi, Dedicatory Volume. A. Kasha and B. Pullman, Editors. Academic Press Inc., New York. 421 pp. 1962.
7. Hackenbrock, C. R.: Ultrastructural Basis for Metabolically Linked Mechanical Activity in Mitochondria. I. Reversible Ultrastructural Changes in Metabolic Steady State in Isolated Liver Mitochondria. *J. Cell. Biol.*, **30**:269, 1966.
8. Hackenbrock, C. R.: Ultrastructural Basis for Metabolically Linked Mechanical Activity in Mitochondria. II. Electron—Transport—Linked Ultrastructural Transformations in Mitochondria. *J. Cell. Biol.*, **37**:345, 1968.
9. Haugaard, N., Hauggard, E. S., Lee, N. H., and Horn, R. S.: Possible Role of Mitochondria in Regulation of Cardiac Contractility. *Fed. Proc.*, **28**:1657, 1969.

General References

Muscatello, U. and Pasquali-Ronchetti, I.: The Relation Between Structure and Function in Mitochondria. Its Relevance in Pathology. In *Pathobiology Annual*. 1972. Series Editor Harry L. Ioachim, M.D. Appleton-Century-Crofts. New York, 1972.

Lehninger, A. L.: *The Mitochondrion*. John Wiley & Sons, New York, 1964.

Needham, D. M.: Biochemistry of Muscular Action. In Bourne, G. H. Ed. *The Structure and Function of Muscle*. Academic Press. New York. Vol. II, p. 55, 1960.

Tapley, D. F., Kimberg, D. V., and Buchanan, J. L.: The Mitochondrion. *N. E. J. Med.*, **276**:1124, 1967.

CHAPTER V

The Sarcoplasmic Reticulum and Relaxation

The interaction between actin and myosin (and hence the contractile event—see Chapter III) stops when calcium is removed from the area of the myofilaments. As soon as this cation is no longer present, the troponin-tropomyosin complex returns to its original configuration and once more blocks the active sites on the thin filaments, making them inaccessible to myosin cross-bridges. The sequential making and breaking of contact between myofilaments stops and sarcomeric shortening or contraction terminates.

Surrounding each sarcomere in the myofiber is a network of complex branching tubules called the sarcoplasmic reticulum (SR) which has a demonstrated ability to pump calcium ions out of the surrounding milieu against a concentration gradient with the consumption of ATP (Figure 1) and (see Figure 2, Chapter I). Because of its ability to transport calcium rapidly (as opposed to mitochondria which also accumulate this cation, but more slowly) the SR is thought to be the subcellular system which is responsible for relaxation in the cell.

The sarcoplasmic reticulum can be isolated from homogenized cardiac or skeletal muscle by ultracentrifugation. Although such preparations are contaminated to some extent by membrane fragments from mitochondria and, to a lesser degree, other cellular components, techniques have improved to the point where a relatively pure suspension of sarcoplasmic reticulum can be obtained. After such treatment, SR membrane is usually almost completely in the form of small, separate round vesicles. These can be prepared for examination in the electron microscope or suspended in media of various ionic composition and the way in which they accumulate and release calcium studied. There are important differences between skeletal and cardiac muscle sarcoplasmic reticulum (Table 1).

Membrane Anatomy and Chemical Composition:

The outer surface of the sarcoplasmic reticular vesicle has a fringe of 30-40 Å particles on its surface (1). Their function is not known, but they may be part of the calcium transport mechanism in the membrane. Skeletal muscle sarcoplasmic reticulum has an additional structural feature—there are 80-90 Å units in the interior of the membrane which are postulated to be ATPases and provide the energy necessary for calcium transport (2).

The SR membrane is, like all others, essentially a lipoprotein. Its major component, however, is protein about 40% of which is a right-handed α-helix and which contains an unusual abundance of active sites. As Mommaerts has pointed out, this multiplicity of active sites is congruent with the necessity to transport relatively massive amounts of calcium over short periods of time (3). Both the ATPase and Ca^{++} transporting activity of the SR membrane, at least in the case of skeletal muscle, are destroyed if the phospholipid (specifically, lecithin) is

75

Figure 1. *This micrograph shows a fragment of the sarcoplasmic reticulum which surrounds the sarcomere in an enveloping sleeve of branching tubules. SR = sarcoplasmic reticulum. Compare to Figure 2, Chapter 1. (x 53,333).*

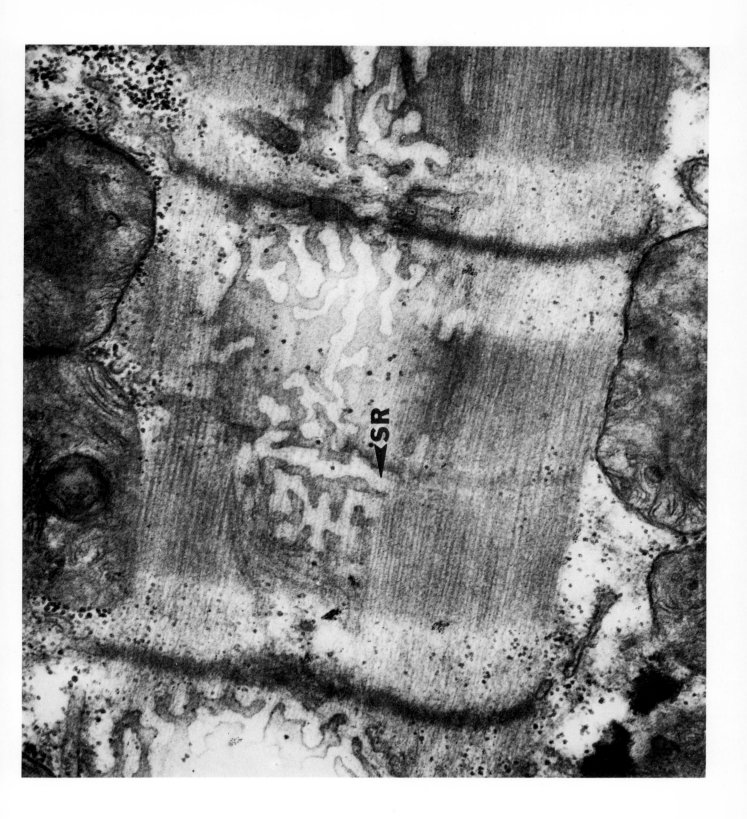

Figure 2. *This fragment of a ventricular cell shows both diadic and triadic units; the lateral sacs of the sarcoplasmic reticulum (LS) come into close apposition with the much larger vesicle which is a portion of the transverse tubular system (T). The amorphous substance in the T-vesicle is the perimembranous component of the sarcolemma (see Chapter II) and is a normal finding in electron micrographs of cells with a transverse tubular system. (x 46,666).*

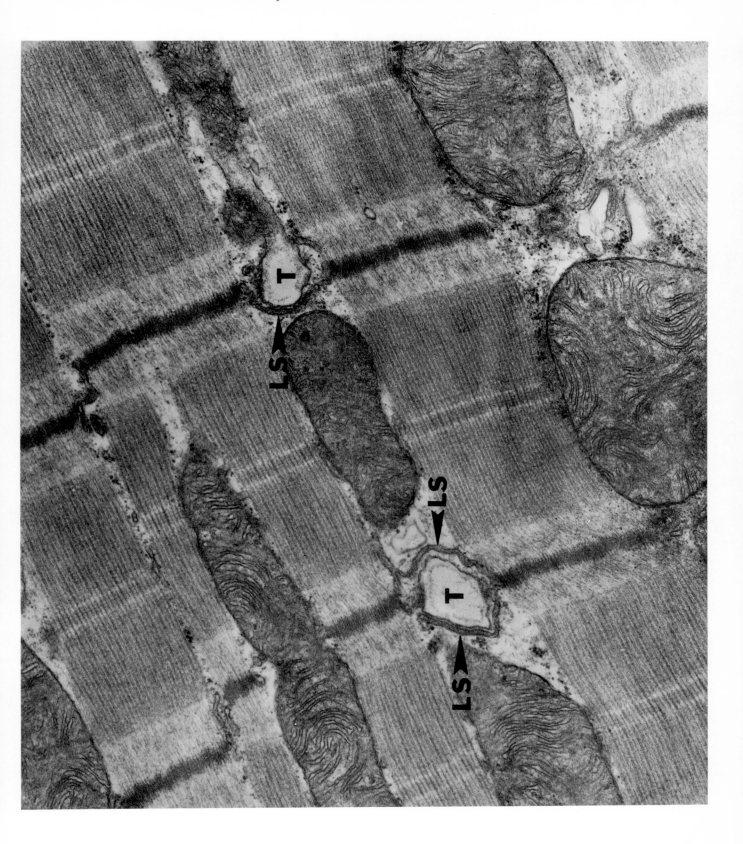

TABLE 1.
DIFFERENCES BETWEEN CARDIAC AND SKELETAL SARCOPLASMIC RETICULUM

	SKELETAL SR	CARDIAC SR
Membrane Characteristics	30-40 Å particulate fringe 80 Å subunits within the membrane are probably ATPase.	30-40 Å particulate fringe — may represent a carrier involved in Ca^{++} transport. No 80 Å subunits in membrane.
Energy Supply	ATP or CTP support relaxation	ATP specific.
Role of Lateral Sac in Excitation-Contraction Coupling	Lateral sacs supply calcium for excitation-contraction coupling.	Unknown; perimembrane calcium may prompt calcium release from lateral sac for distribution of this cation to the area of the myofilaments.
Rate of Ca^{++} Binding	SR of white skeletal muscle binds calcium fastest; red skeletal muscle of SR binds calcium slowly.	Speed of calcium binding intermediate between that of white and red skeletal muscle sarcoplasmic reticulum.
Morphology (Figure 3)	Central cisterna. Lateral sacs large.	No central cisterna. Much smaller lateral sacs.

removed from the membrane. This may be due to the fact, however, that the lipid components of the membrane serve primarily to align the protein constituents correctly so their function can be maintained and not to any primary role of the lipid as either a carrier molecule or an ATPase.

Mechanism of Calcium Transport

The exact way in which the sarcoplasmic reticulum transports calcium from the environment is not known: whether a carrier molecule is involved, whether calcium is exchanged for another ion in the process of transport, whether it is actively bound to the membrane or transported into the lumen of the tubule where it is combined with an anion, are all things we do not know. In vitro, active binding (that is, a process requiring ATP) to the membrane occurs and suggests that phosphorylization of the carrier molecule is necessary for calcium accumulation. If oxalate is added to the milieu, calcium is transported across the membrane and combines with the oxalate in the vescicle's interior, where it is stored as the electron-dense salt of calcium oxalate and is visible in the electron microscope. Lanthanum does not replace calcium in the cardiac sarcoplasmic reticular membrane, indicating that calcium is bound at a specific binding site and not held to the membrane by simple electrostatic attraction (4).

The recent work of Repke and Katz indicates that in cardiac SR, there is probably a two-step mechanism of calcium accumulation: the first is by *binding* of Ca++ to high affinity sites on the membrane and the second is by *uptake* of Ca++ via non-facilitated diffusion of this cation (at locations in the membrane other than the binding site) across the membrane: the speed of the latter process is concentration-related and does not demonstrate saturation kinetics (5). Whether there is a substance analogous to oxalate in the SR lumen that traps calcium is, at the moment, unknown.

Several investigators, notably Schwarz and Katz, have calculated from their data on Ca^{++} binding by cardiac vesicles that myocardial sarcoplasmic reticulum is both abundant enough and able to bind calcium rapidly enough so that it certainly could be the subcellular system that achieves relaxation in the cell (6, 7). Others postulate that mitochondria, which also accumulate calcium, are the organelles that effect beat-to-beat relaxation in the cell. The very rapid calcium-binding ability of the SR in comparison to the slower rates at which mitochondria accumulate calcium make the sarcoplasmic reticulum a more likely candidate for this role in the myofiber. Mitochondria may regulate the Ca^{++} levels inside the cell in an important way, however, and in so doing make an important contribution to the control of contractile force in myocardium. Whether they actually do so, and to what extent, remains to be demonstrated, however.

Several factors influence the rate at which the sarcoplasmic reticulum transports calcium. These may be important in the regulation of cellular contractility.

Hydrogen ion concentration, at least in vitro, prompts the release of calcium by SR membranes in skeletal muscle. An increase in H^+ ion concentration has been shown, again in skeletal muscle, vesicles to prompt calcium rebinding by the SR (8).

Intracellular pH has been estimated, on the basis of direct intracellular measurement, to be as high as 7.69 in the depolarized state and as low as 3.25 in the hyperpolarized cell; the change in H^+ ion concentration may be an important mechanism for the control of the SR calcium accumulating ability, enhancing it during depolarization and inhibiting it when the cell is in a resting state (8).

Inorganic phosphate concentration also has in vitro a regulatory effect on cardiac SR calcium uptake. Inorganic phosphate (P_i) in the medium accelerates calcium accumulation by the vesicles (9). This may be an important feedback mechanism in vivo, whereby the inorganic phosphate (P_i) produced from the ATP split during contraction acts on the adjacent sarcotubular network to stimulate rates of calcium transport and hence facilitate rapid sarcomeric relaxation.

The Sarcoplasmic Reticulum and Excitation—Contraction Coupling

The sarcoplasmic reticular membrane not only binds calcium, it releases it. There are specialized areas of the sarcoplasmic reticular system called lateral sacs. These lie closely approximated in the cell to the sarcolemma and its derivatives, the transverse tubular system and the intercalated disc (Figures, 2, 3). Although the morphology of the SR differs somewhat between skeletal and cardiac muscle (Figure 4) the lateral sacs in both types of sarcoplasmic reticulum are depots for large concentrations of calcium ion. Electron dense deposits of calcium antimonate have been produced and visualized within the lateral sacs of cardiac muscle perfused with potassium antimonate solution (Figure 5), (10). At least in skeletal muscle, it is clear that the depolarizing impulse initiated at the sarcolemma, is propagated swiftly throughout the entire substance of the myofiber over the transverse tubular membrane and prompts Ca^{++} release at the level of each sarcomere from the lateral sacs (see Chapter II, the transverse tubular system).

As A. V. Hill has pointed out, the short time between excitation and the contractile event in skeletal muscle requires that calcium be released virtually simultaneously at all levels of the cell in response to depolarization (11). In cardiac muscle, however, the time between depolarization and the contractile event is much longer (about 300 msec.) than in skeletal muscle. Calcium diffuses

Figures 3 and 4. *These sketches show the differences in morphology between cardiac and skeletal sarcoplasmic reticulum. The lateral sacs are not of the same dimension and there is a central fenestrated cisterna in skeletal sarcoplasmic reticulum. The differences in diadic and triadic configurations in the two result from these variations. Note also the difference in the size of the transverse tubule; it is of much smaller diameter in skeletal than in cardiac muscle.*

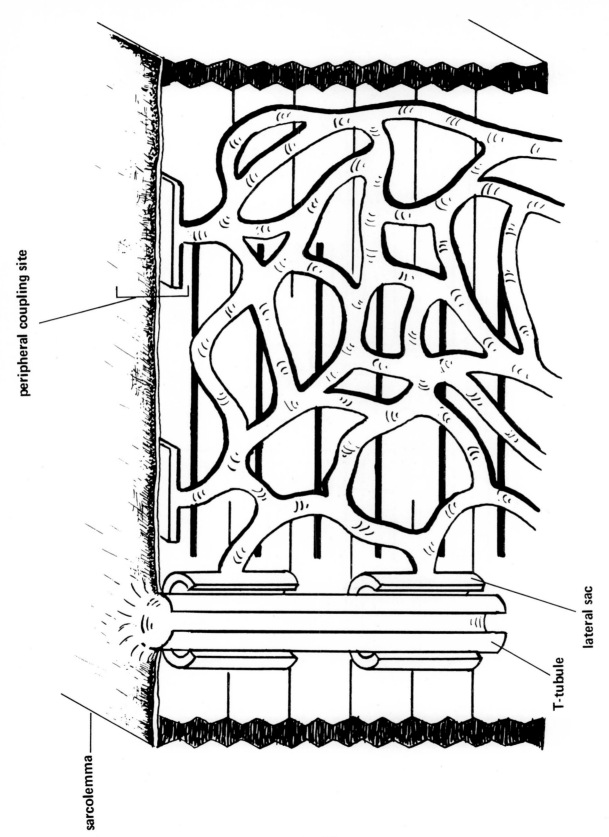

peripheral coupling site

sarcolemma

lateral sac

T-tubule

3. Cardiac Muscle Sarcoplasmic Reticulum

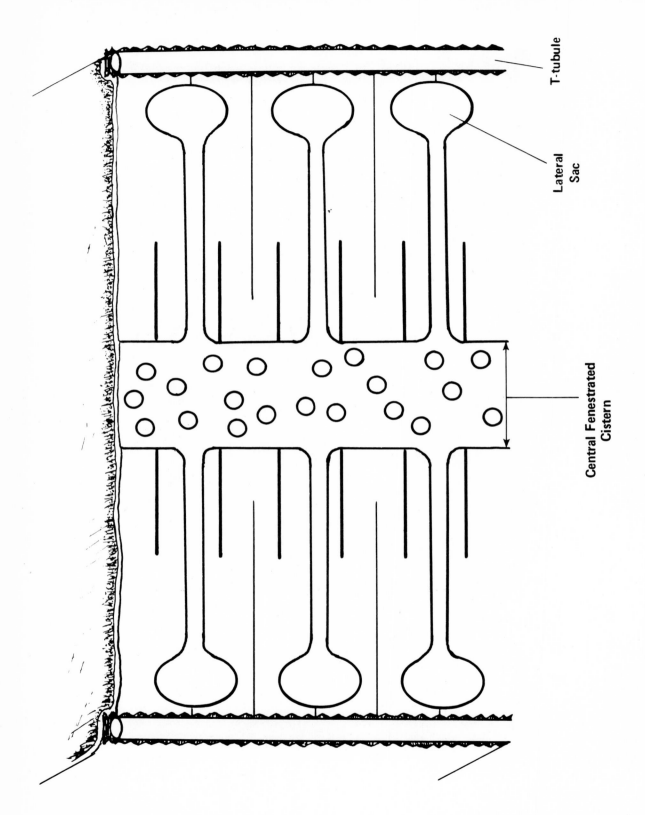

T-tubule

Lateral Sac

Central Fenestrated Cistern

4. Skeletal Muscle Sarcoplasmic Reticulum

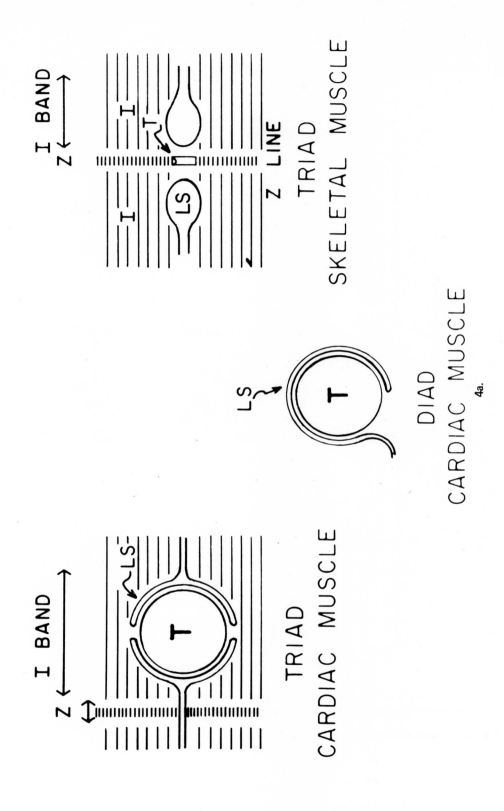

Figure 5. *This electron micrograph shows a triad in cardiac tissue. Note that the lateral sacs contain a dense precipitate of calcium antimonate (arrows), indicating that there is an abundance of this cation (Ca^{++}) in the lateral sacs of cardiac muscle. (x 173,257).*

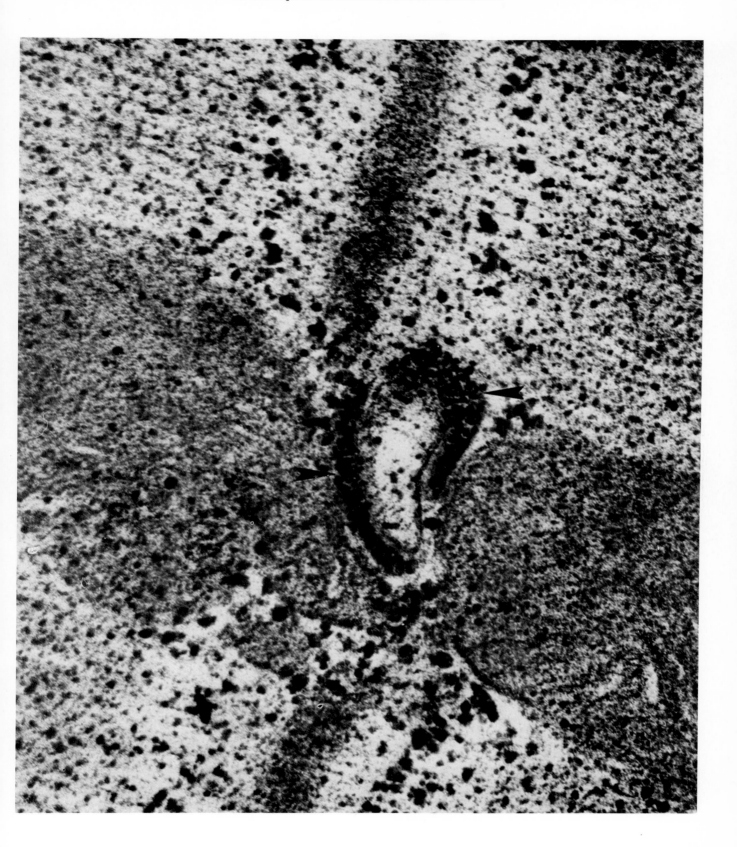

at a rate of 1 micron per millisecond through myoplasm. The diameter of the myofiber is small enough (the average diameter of ventricular cell is 10-15μ) to allow for calcium to penetrate the entire thickness of the cell from the surface of the myofiber by the process of simple diffusion. There is no theoretical need, therefore, for an anatomic substrate such as the triad where depolarization prompts coupling calcium release from the lateral sacs at multiple levels of the myofiber.

The definitive experiment to test the role of the T system in excitation-contraction coupling in cardiac tissue would, of course, be to destroy it and to measure the effect of such a loss on the ability of the cell to contract in response to excitation. Although, as Howell has demonstrated (12), such selective destruction of the T system is possible in skeletal muscle (where the cell so treated is uncoupled; it no longer responds with contraction to an exciting impulse, although it continues to generate an action potential), cardiac T-system is invulnerable to glycerol and hypertonic solution and remains quite intact after such treatment (13). This difference in response between skeletal and cardiac muscle transverse tubular systems serves to highlight further the probability that there are fundamental differences between the systems in the two types of muscle (Figure 4, Table 1).

It is probable that excitation-contraction coupling in cardiac tissue is effected (as we have discussed in Chapter II) by calcium ion released from the perimembrane, and the function of the calcium ion in the lateral sacs of cardiac SR is really not demonstrated. It may be simply a storage depot for calcium in the myofiber to which intracellular Ca++ is confined, inactive, until it can be extruded from the cell into the extracellular space. It may also function, by virtue of its ability to accumulate and release calcium, to control the permeability characteristics of the membranes to which it is approximated, not only the T-tubular membrane, but the sarcolemma and the intercalated disc.

A substantial number of investigators, however, feel that cardiac SR (specifically, the membrane of the lateral sacs) *is* the source of excitation-contraction calcium in the myofiber as it is in skeletal muscle. Palmer and Posey, for example, have shown that Na$^+$ ion produces the release of a certain fraction of calcium bound and transported by cardiac SR, and suggest that the sodium entering the cell at the moment of depolarization engenders calcium release from the membrane of the lateral sac, thus initiating contraction (14).

It may be that the truth is somewhere between the two positions, and that perimembrane calcium entering the cell at the time of depolarization replaces the calcium on the lateral sac membrane, which in turn is released to the myofilaments and engenders the contractile event.

Drugs and the Sarcoplasmic Reticulum

Although the effect of drugs on the sarcotubular system has been rather extensively studied in skeletal muscle, we have not accumulated as much data about the pharmacology of cardiac reticulum. Quinidine inhibits cardiac SR calcium uptake. Catecholamines, which augment calcium influx into the cell during the plateau phase of the action potential, produces increased systolic force in the cell. They may effect this either by increasing calcium released from an internal storage site in the cell *or* they may enhance the receptivity of the receptor sites to calcium; which is not known. Adrenergic blocking agents such as propanalol depress calcium uptake by cardiac SR. Caffeine in low concentrations increases the systolic force generated by the cell and in high concentrations, retards the rate of relaxation in the myofiber by retarding calcium uptake by the sarcoplasmic reticulum. Similarly, amytal inhibits calcium uptake by the SR; digitalis reverses this inhibition. Digitalis also reverses the depressed calcium uptake exhibited by the SR of the failing myocardium. There are conflicting data about the effect of digitalis on normal, untreated vesicles in the heart; some investigators find that *in vitro* this drug enhances the amount of calcium transported by the SR. Since, however, digitalis is almost certainly restricted to the extracellular compartment in myocardium, producing an effect at the sarcolemma, *in vitro* experiments with digitalis and isolated vesicles are not necessarily relevant to the situation in the intact animal. Schwartz, who has done extensive and careful work with cardiac SR, found no effect of digitalis on normal vesicles (15). He and his co-workers suggest that the alleged effect of digitalis on SR calcium binding and exchange is due to the presence of Na^+-K^+ stimulated ATPase in the preparation; possibly a sarcolemmal contaminant. The method of preparation of cardiac vesicles is crucial; often the vesicles are contaminated by mitochondrial and sarcolemmal membrane fragments and careful evaluation of the purity of the preparation is in order when evaluating its characteristics.

Table 2 summarizes some of the effects of drugs on the calcium-accumulating ability of sarcotubular vesicles isolated from both cardiac and skeletal muscles. It must be emphasized that the pharmacologic effects of the drugs on myocardial contractility are not necessarily the consequence of their action on the sarcoplasmic reticulum. Those investigators who attribute diminished force development by heart muscle to an effect on the sarcoplasmic reticulum make the assumption that myocardial contractility is a direct consequence of the intracellular calcium content of the myofiber, which, in turn, is under the exclusive control of the sarcoplasmic reticulum. This is probably not the case: mitochondrial control of the calcium content of the sarcoplasm is an important factor in the maintenance of the intracellular milieu; there are even data showing that oligomycin, which inhibits Ca^{++} uptake by the mitochondria, prevents effective relaxation of the heart between each beat (16). Mitochondria contain the highest fraction of calcium in the heart and, like the sarcoplasic reticulum, are stimulated to take up calcium by P_i. This, together with their abundance and proximity to the myofilaments, have led some workers to feel that they, and not the sarcotubular system, are the subcellular organelles which achieve beat-to-beat relaxation in the heart. Evidence for this hypothesis is not incontrovertible for the intact heart at this time, however.

There are important differences in the way the mitochondria and the sarcotubular system handle calcium; these are summarized in Table 3.

The Sarcoplasmic Reticulum in Pathologic States

There are data which suggest that in certain pathologic conditions there is dysfunction of the sarcoplasmic reticulum in that its ability to accumulate calcium is depressed. For example, Schwarz has shown a depression of calcium accumulating and releasing ability in SR isolated from failing myocardium (17). Similarly, Lee has demonstrated that ischemia for a ninety minute period produces irreversible damage to the capacity of cardiac vesicles to take up calcium;

TABLE 2
THE EFFECT OF DRUGS ON THE SARCOPLASMIC RETICULUM

Drug	Type of Muscle Studied	Action on Isolated SR Vesicle and Proposed Mechanism for Effect on Myocardial Function	Effect on Myocardial Function
Catecholamines	Cardiac	Augments slow inward calcium current occurring during plateau of action potential. (Does this calcium prompt release of calcium in an internal cellular storage site such as the sarcoplasmic reticulum?)	Increases systolic force generated by muscle.
Adrenergic Blocking Agents (Propanalol)	Cardiac	Depress ability of SR to accumulate calcium—this may result in an eventual decrease in intracellular calcium.	Diminishes cardiac contractility.
Digitalis	Cardiac	No effect on purified preparation.	Enhanced inotropism is probably entirely the consequence of an effect at the sarcolemma and not within the cell in the intact animal.
Quinidine	Cardiac and skeletal.	Depresses calcium accumulation by SR vesicles.	In low concentrations potentiates myocardial contractility; in higher concentrations, depresses it. In low concentrations in skeletal muscle, quinidine potentiates twitch tension, in higher concentrations, causes contracture: relaxing ability of SR is destroyed.
Barbiturates	Cardiac	Depresses calcium accumulating ability of SR vesicles.	Depression of myocardial contractility
Caffeine	Skeletal	Low concentrations prompt release of calcium from the sarcoplasmic reticulum.	Increases systolic force of twitch in skeletal muscle. (A well-demonstrated direct effect on the sarcoplasmic reticulum.)
Anions	Cardiac	High concentrations depress calcium uptake by SR.	Retard rate of relaxation in the muscle.
	Skeletal	Substitution of SCN^-, I^-, $NO3^-$ for Cl^- in perfusate causes depressed SR uptake of calcium.	Effect on intact muscle function unknown.
Cations (Zn^{++})	Cardiac	Zinc depresses calcium uptake of SR.	Depresses myocardial contractility; this may be due to a blockade of extracellular calcium from entering the cell, however.

after 60 minutes, SR function returns to normal if the coronary circulation is restored (18). Skeletal muscle in thyrotoxic hypokalemic periodic paralysis has remarkably enlarged lateral sacs in the sarcotubular system (19); cardiac muscle has not been studied in this disorder. How diminished calcium uptake or release by the sarcoplasmic reticulum contributes to depressed myocardial contractility (if at all) is not readily apparent; in cardiac tissue it is not clear that SR calcium is functional in excitation—contraction coupling. Theoretically a depressed ability of the SR to accumulate calcium ought to result in impaired relaxation of muscle, or a rise in diastolic tension. So, although the effect of drugs on the SR and the Ca++ accumulating ability of the myocardium have been studied to a certain extent, the actual role sarcoplasmic reticular dysfunction plays in the decompensated or diseased myocardium remains unclear.

TABLE 3
DIFFERENCES BETWEEN MITOCHONDRIA AND SARCOPLASMIC RETICULAR CALCIUM UPTAKE

MITOCHONDRIA	SARCOPLASMIC RETICULUM
Rate of Ca^{++} uptake increases with calcium concentrations in the range of $10^{-5} - 3 \times 10^{-3}$ M.	No influence of Ca^{++} concentration on rate of uptake.
Somewhat unstable with respect to changes in temperature and ionic concentration.	Ca^{++} uptake preserved after 30 days of freezing at $-20°$ F.
Oligomycin, sodium azide or 2-4 dinitrophenol inhibit Ca^{++} uptake.	No inhibition of Ca^{++} uptake by these substances.
Ca^{++} uptake *not* stimulated by oxalate.	Ca^{++} uptake stimulated by oxalate.
ATP only energy supply (very specific for this).	ATP, CTP, GTP, or ITP can all be utilized.

Specific References

1. Baskin, R. J. and Deamer, D. W.: Comparative Ultrastructure and Calcium Transport in Heart and Skeletal Muscle Microsomes. *J. Cell. Biol.*, 43:610, 1969.
2. Deamer, D. W. and Baskin, R. J.: Ultrastructure of Sarcoplasmic Reticulum Preparations. *J. Cell. Biol.*, 42:296, 1969.
3. Mommaerts, W. H. F. M.: Conformational Studies on the Membrane Protein of Sarcotubular Vesicles. *Proc. Natl. Acad. Sci.*, 58:2476, 1967.
4. Entman, M. L., Hansen, J. L., and Cook, J. W. Jr.: Calcium Metabolism in Cardiac Microsomes Incubated with Lanthanum Ion. *Biochem. Biophys. Res. Comm.*, 35:258, 1969.
5. Repke, D. and Katz, A. M.: Calcium-binding and Calcium Uptake by Cardiac Microsomes: A Kinetic Analysis. *J. Mol. Cell Cardiol.*, 4:401, 1972.
6. Harigaya, S. and Schwartz, A.: Rate of Calcium Binding and Uptake in Normal Animal and Failing Human Cardiac Muscle. *Circ. Res.*, 25:781, 1969.
7. Katz, A. M. and Repke, D.: Quantitative Aspects of Dog Cardiac Microsomal Calcium Binding and Calcium Uptake. *Circ. Res.*, 21:153, 1967.

8. Nakamaru, Y. and Schwartz, A.: The Influence of Hydrogen Ion Concentration on Calcium Binding and Release by Skeletal Muscle Sarcoplasmic Reticulum. *J. Gen. Physiol.*, **59**:22, 1972.

9. Lee, K. S.: Present Status of Cardiac Relaxing Factor. *Fed. Proc.* 24:1432, 1965.

10. Legato, M. J.: Subcellular Localization of Calcium Ion in Mammalian Myocardium. *J. Cell. Biol.*, **41**:401, 1969.

11. Hill, A. V.: On the Time Required for Diffusion and Its Relations to Processes in Muscle. *Proc. Roy. Soc. (London)*, Series B 135:446, 1948.

12. Howell, J. N. and Jenden, D. J.: T-Tubules of Skeletal Muscle: Morphological Alterations Which Interrupt Excitation-Contraction Coupling. *Fed. Proc. FASEB.*, **26**:553, 1967.

13. Niemeyer, G. and Forssman, W. G.: Comparison of Glycerol Treatment in Frog Skeletal Muscle and Mammalian Heart. *J. Cell. Biol.*, **50**:288, 1971.

14. Palmer, R. F. and Posey, V.: Ion Effects on Calcium Accumulation by Cardiac Sarcoplasmic Reticulum. *J. Gen. Physiol.*, **50**:2085, 1967.

15. Entman, M., Allen, J. C., and Schwartz, A.: Calcium—Interaction in a "Microsomal" Membrane Fraction Containing Na^+, K^+- ATPase Activity and Calcium Binding Activity. *J. Mol. Cell. Cardiol.*, 4:435, 1972.

16. Fehmers, M. C. O.: *Intracellular Ca^{++} en de Werking van Hartspier*. Academic Thesis, Amsterdam: Univ. Amsterdam, Hollandia. Offset druk Kerij, 1968.

17. Harigaya, S. and Schwartz, A.: Rate of Calcium Binding and Uptake in Normal Animal and Failing Human Cardiac Muscle. Membrane Vesicles (relaxing system) and Mitochondria. *Circ. Res.*, **25**:781, 1969.

18. Lee, K. S., Ladinsky, H., and Stukey, J. H.: Decreased Ca^{2+} Uptake by Sarcoplasmic Reticulum After Coronary Artery Occlusion for 60 and 90 Minutes. *Circ. Res.*, 21:439, 1967.

19. Schutta, H. S. and Armitage, J. L.: The Sarcoplasmic Reticulum in Thyrotoxic Hypokalemic Periodic Paralysis. *Metabolism*, 18:81, 1969.

General References

Gergely, J. et. al.: Physiology Symposium. The Relaxing Factor of Muscle. *Fed. Proc.*, **23**:885, Sept.-Oct. 1964.

Lee, K. S. Present Status of Cardiac Relaxing Factor. *Fed. Proc.*, 24:1432, 1965.

CHAPTER VI

Myocardial Growth and Hypertrophy: The Cell in Congestive Heart Failure and the Mechanism of Digitalis Action

The myocardial cell in adult life does not divide and multiply. The number of cells in the heart is fixed after early post-natal life, although mitosis continues for a short time after birth. Cardiac hypertrophy, therefore, is the consequence of the enlargement of already existing myofibers and of the proliferation of non-muscular elements of the myocardium: connective tissue and endothelial cells.

Transcription and Translation

The nucleus is, as in all cells, the depot of genetic information in the myofiber. Nuclear chromosomes are composed of desoxyribonucleic acid (DNA), a molecule consisting of two parallel strands of nucleotides joined to one another via their ribose moieties. In mitosis, when the cell divides, the strands of DNA separate, and one each is distributed to two daughter cells. Each single strand then serves as the template for the assembly of a second strand of nucleotides to which it is joined and the chromosome is completed.

Once the genetic information of the cell is complete, DNA instructs the formation of new proteins in the cell. This process continues for the life of the cell, which, in the case of the myofiber, extends for the lifetime of the animal. Nuclear DNA instructs the formation of messenger RNA (mRNA), which is a strand of riboneucleic acid that copies the base sequence of one of the two strands of DNA in the process known as *transcription*. Messenger RNA is exported from the nucleus, probably via the nuclear-cytoplasmic bridges called the nuclear pores (Figures 1, 2, 3). In the cytoplasm, RNA instructs the assembly of new proteins in conjunction with two other entities: small particles called ribosomes and complexes of an amino acid attached to another type of RNA called transfer RNA (tRNA). This is the process known as *translation*.

Ribosomes are particles containing a unique type of RNA, so-called ribosomal RNA (rRNA). The precursors of this RNA come from the nucleolus of the cell. Ribosomes have two components—a large 50S and a smaller 30S moiety. The two ribosomal fragments align themselves along the thin linear strand of mRNA, one on each side, and an amino acid, combined with its specific tRNA, attaches to the 30S component of the ribosome (Figure 4). From there it is transferred to the 50S component. The ribosome then moves along the mRNA in steps of three nucleotides, adding a new amino acid to its growing peptide chain at each step.

Figure 1. *This micrograph shows sections of three atrial cells. The nucleus (N) is bound by a double membrane. Note the peripherally clumped chromatin (Ch) just under the inner membrane of the nucleus. The nuclear pole (at the end of the nucleus) contains the Golgi apparatus (GA), mitochondria, (M) glycogen (G) and atrial granules (AG). (x 18,666).*

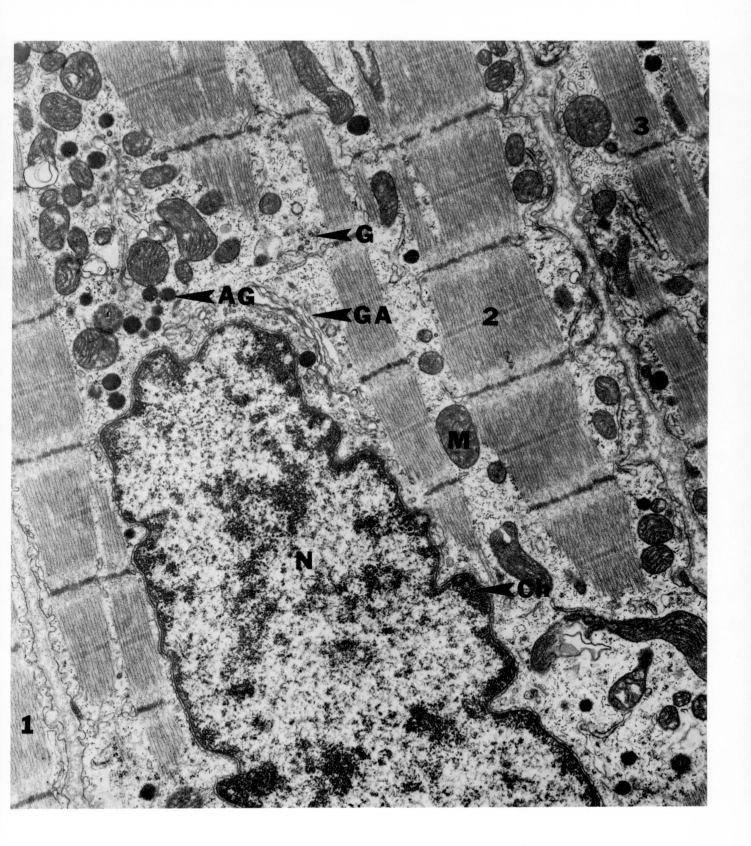

Figure 2. *This illustrates the nuclear-cytoplasmic bridges called nuclear pores (NP) in cross-section. (See text). (x 37,332).*

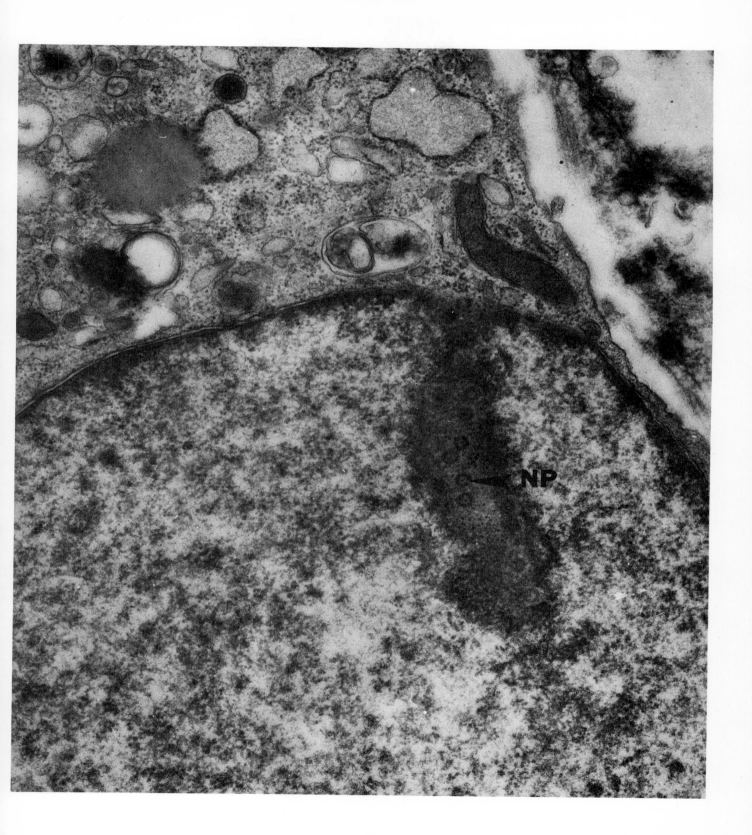

Figure 3. *This micrograph shows the continuity of Golgi apparatus with the outer nuclear membrane and shows the nuclear pore (NP) in longitudinal section. Note the electron-dense line crossing the nuclear pore at its center; this corresponds to the dark material circling the pore in Figure 2, where the pore is seen in cross section. (x 68,442).*

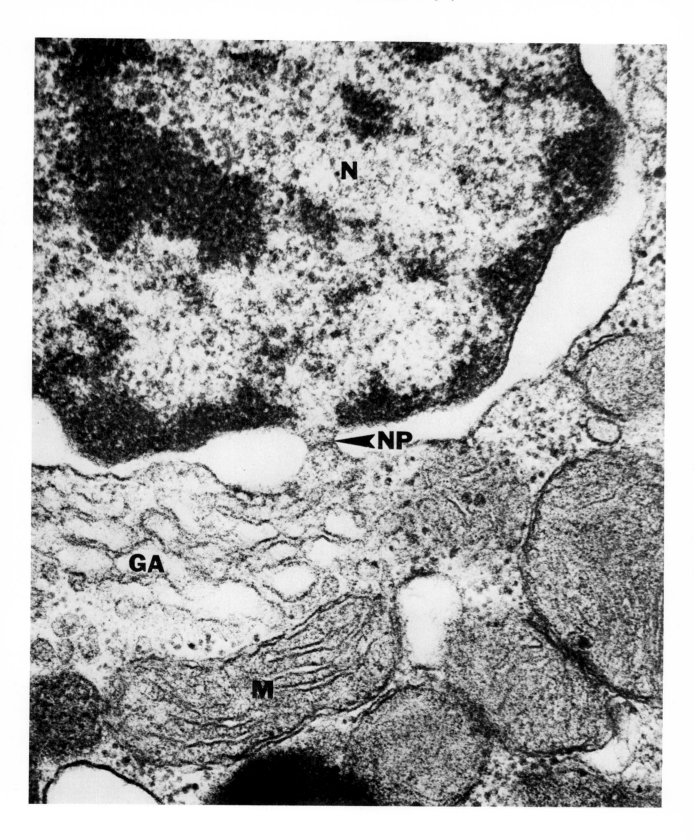

Figure 4. *This is a summary of the steps involved in the process of translation and transcription.*

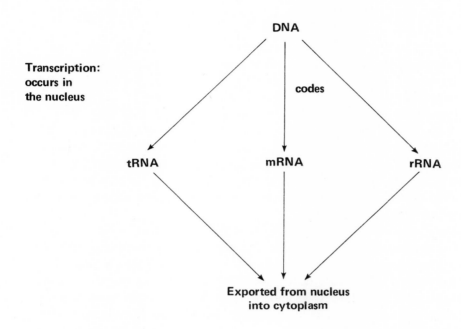

occurs in
the nucleus

Translation:
occurs in
the cytoplasm

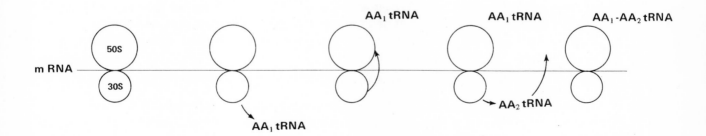

Portion of a Polyribosome

Transcription and Translation

Guanidine triphosphate (GTP) supplies the energy for the addition of the amino acids to the chain. With each addition, the tRNA of the previously added complex is removed. Aggregates of 3-10 ribosomes are necessary for the synthesis of one protein; such groups of ribosomes are called *polyribosomes* (Figure 5).

Messenger RNA serves as a template for many ribosomes at one time; each ribosome bears a growing polypeptide chain as it moves along the mRNA in steps of three nucleotides. Messenger RNA has a transient existence in the cell and does not accumulate.

Each of the twenty amino acids has one or more specific tRNA's. All tRNA's have triple sequences of basis (or codons) which are complimentary and opposite to that of the triple unit of mRNA. Transfer RNA, like mRNA, is coded by DNA and must also be manufactured in and exported from the nucleus.

Ribosomes themselves have two different types of still a different type of RNA—one kind is 16.35 S rRNA and is a component of the 30S moiety of the ribosome. It has a molecular weight of 5.6×10^5. The other is a 23.5 S rRNA, with a molecular weight of 1.1×10^6. The ribosomal particles are electron dense and can be seen in the electron microscope as dark, round particles very similar to glycogen particles. They are either loose in the cytoplasm or aligned on the outside of endoplasmic reticular tubules.

The endoplasmic reticulum has its origin in and is contiguous with the outer membrane of the nucleus, beginning as the complex folding system of tubules called the Golgi apparatus (Figures 1, 3). When ribosomal particles are aligned on the outer aspect of the endoplasmic reticulum (ER), the tubular system is called rough endoplasmic reticulum (RER) (Figures 6, 7). In cells where new protein, either for purposes of growth or repair, is being made at rapid or increased rates, rough endoplasmic reticulum is abundant. It is most prominent at the nuclear poles, but can also be seen in enlarging cells out in the periphery of the cell, although this is an unusual finding in the adult myofiber. RER can be observed in the area of damage in a myofiber, in the cells of young animals who are actively growing and increasing their heart size, and in rapidly hypertrophying tissue.

Loose, free ribosomal particles are difficult to tell from glycogen granules, and special techniques are needed to distinguish between them. Glycogen in myocardial cells is often arranged in clumps or "rosettes," however; ribosomes lie randomly arranged unless they are aggregated in a double row along the thin threads of mRNA. These are special groups of ribosomes, the polyribosomes, and it is on them, as we have said, that polypeptide chains are being assembled into proteins.

Mechanisms of Sarcomerogenesis and Mitochondrial Proliferation

The increase in cell size of the post-natal hypertrophied or growing heart is due to the multiplication of two cellular components; the sarcomeres, and the mitochondria. The method by which new sarcomeres are produced in the myocardium is of special interest in our laboratory. It became clear from observations we made of myocardial cells grown in tissue culture that myofilaments were produced in association with abundant masses of Z substance (1). In fact, it soon became apparent that there was much more Z substance in the myoblast than existed in the adult cell (Figure 8). Z substance, therefore, is either consumed or transformed as the cell matures. The Z substance of these early cells was associated with a homogenous group of filaments which were thinner than myosin but more electron dense than finished sarcomeric thin filaments (Figure 9). We called them "primary myofilaments" and were interested to see that (1) they preceded the appearance of thick and thin filaments in finished sarcomeres and (2) that they seemed to be associated closely with those fragments of thin and thick filaments that had appeared and were being made into sarcomeres. Indeed finished thick and thin filaments often seemed to be "spinning off" a parent unit of Z substance which had differentiated in its mid-portion into primary myofilaments.

From the tissue culture preparation we turned to the examination of specimens from growing or hypertrophying human and dog myocardium (2). Sarcomerogenesis also occurs in association with proliferation of Z substance in these myofibers, wherever Z substance is present, either in sarcomeres or at the intercalated disc. Z substance also accumulates at the cell periphery, just under the plasma membrane of the sarcolemma; some investigators have even suggested that Z substance is a membranous derivative because of this association (3).

When Z substance proliferates in subsarcolemmal Z bands, it extends an arm of Z substance in either direction just under the cell membrane (Figure 10). Often Z substance is increasing at the other end of the same sarcomere, and the arms of adjacent Z bands meet, joining to form a sub-sarcolemmal arch (Figure 11). If such areas are examined in the electron microscope, one can see that they are composed of a homogeneous group of filaments, thinner than the sarcomeric thick filament but less electron dense than the thin filament. From this group of filaments, which we have called "primary myofilaments," fragments of thick and thin filaments can be seen spinning off the amassed Z substance, and being laid down in register with the thick and thin filaments in the subjacent sarcomere. In this manner, the height of the sarcomere is increasing and with it, the cell's diameter.

Deep within the cell, Z substance proliferation and differentiation also is apparent. This begins as a subtle, fusiform swelling of Z bands (Figure 12 a and b), but at its maximum is a complexly contoured mass of Z substance remarkable for its bilateral symmetry (Figure 13 a and b). It is at its widest; the size of a single sarcomere (about 2.0 microns in diameter) (Figure 14).

The polarity of the Z band, as we have discussed in Chapter III, is reversed in the midline; this allows the polarized thin filaments to be aligned in opposite senses on either side of the Z bands, thus insuring the correct direction of movement of thin filaments during the contractile event. It would seem then, that the proliferation of Z substance begins at the center and proceeds at exactly the same rate in opposite directions at any given level of the Z band. This explains the remarkable symmetry of the component halves of the hypertrophied mass of Z substance. The Z material then begins to differentiate, again in the midline, and primary myofilaments begin to be apparent in the center of these masses (Figure 15). Differentiation of Z substance progresses and spinning off of thick and thin filaments begins from the parent unit, the finished units being laid down from above and below the primary myofilaments. If the primary myofilaments are reversed in polarity in the midline, as is the parent Z substance, this would insure the reversal of polarity necessary in the finished sarcomeric filaments. Of interest is the fact that although we saw thin filaments of 1μ, the length of a mature thin filament, in association with these masses of Z material, we saw only thick filaments of half the length (0.75μ) of the finished myosin filament (about 1.5μ) coming from opposite ends of the collection of primary myofilaments.

Figure 5. *This is a portion of a rat ventricular cell grown in tissue culture which contains the double chain of ribosomes on which the synthesis of new proteins is taking place in the cell. Such an aggregation is called a polyribosome (PR). (x 78,545).*

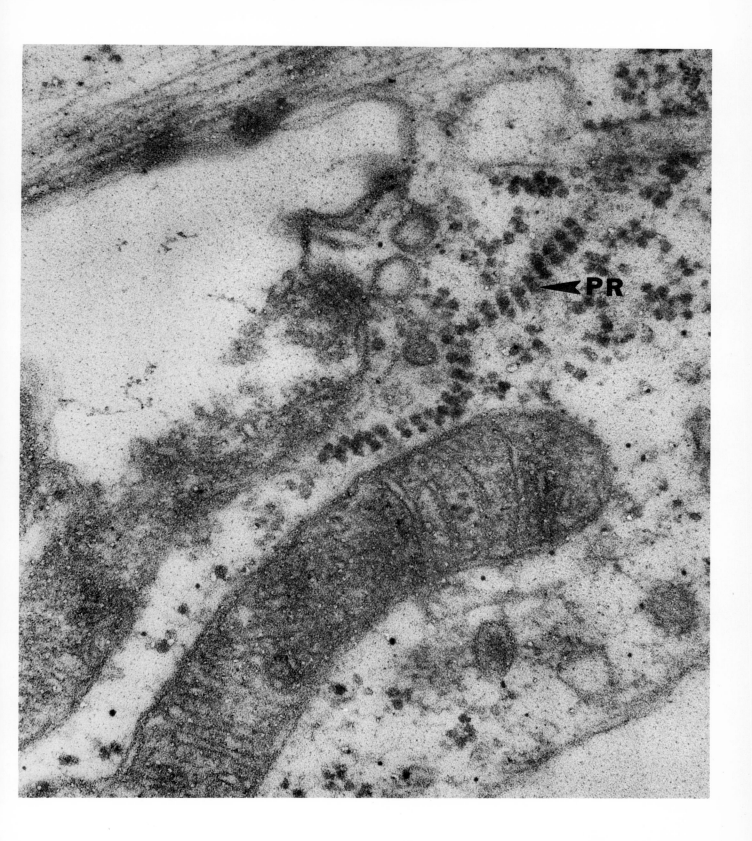

Figure 6. *This is a fragment of a cell in the area of the nucleus where ribosomes are beginning to align themselves along the outer aspect of the reticular membrane to form "rough endoplasmic reticulum" (RER). They are transported along the reticular network to the places in the cell where new protein synthesis is required. (x 109,333).*

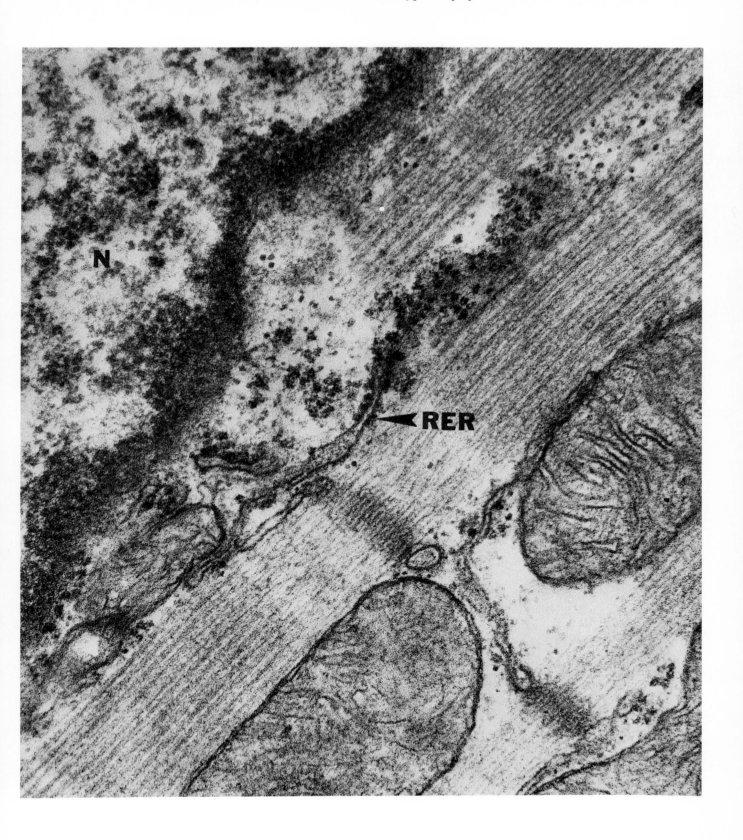

Figure 7. *This is high power view of a portion of a two-day old rat ventricular cell grown in tissue culture which shows fragments of rough endoplasmic reticulum (arrows) and ribosomes loose in the cytoplasm (circle). (x 90,000).*

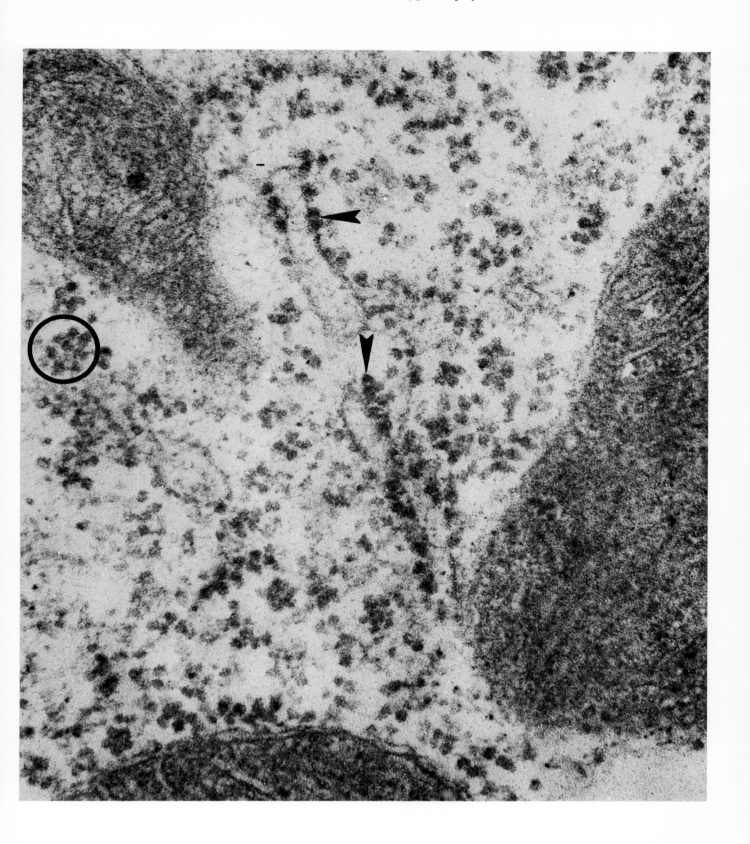

Figure 8. *This portion of a rat ventricular cell grown in tissue culture shows developing sarcomeric units in association with clumps of Z substance (Z). The amount of Z substance in the young myoblast is much more than that in the adult myofiber. (x 31,059).*

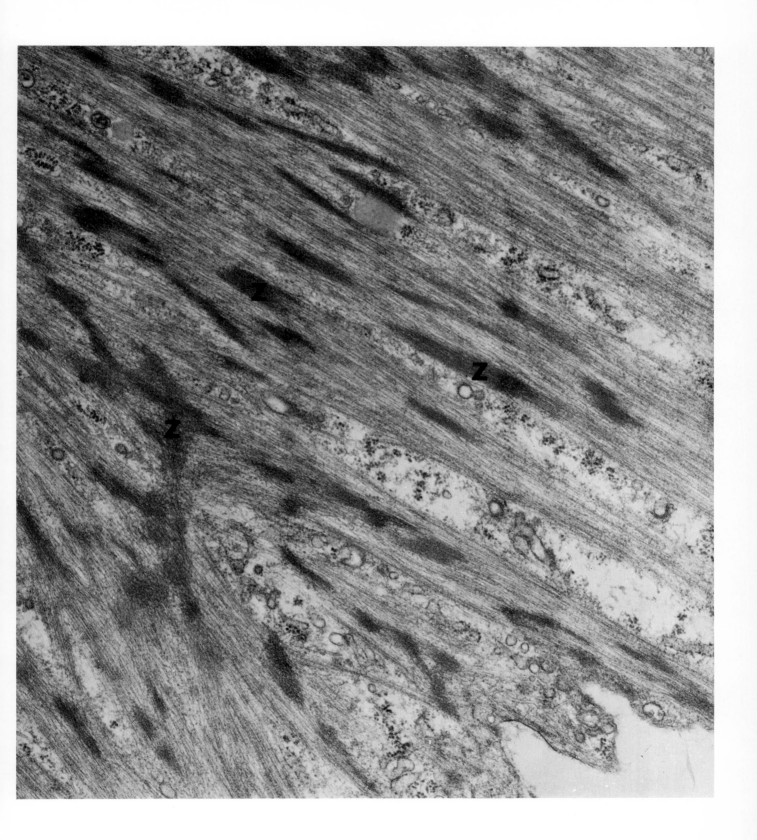

Figure 9. *Under the sarcolemma of this myoblast are clustered primary myofilaments (arrows), a homogeneous group of primitive myofilaments which are the first to appear in the cell (see text). ECS = extracellular space. PM = perimembrance. (x 70,000).*

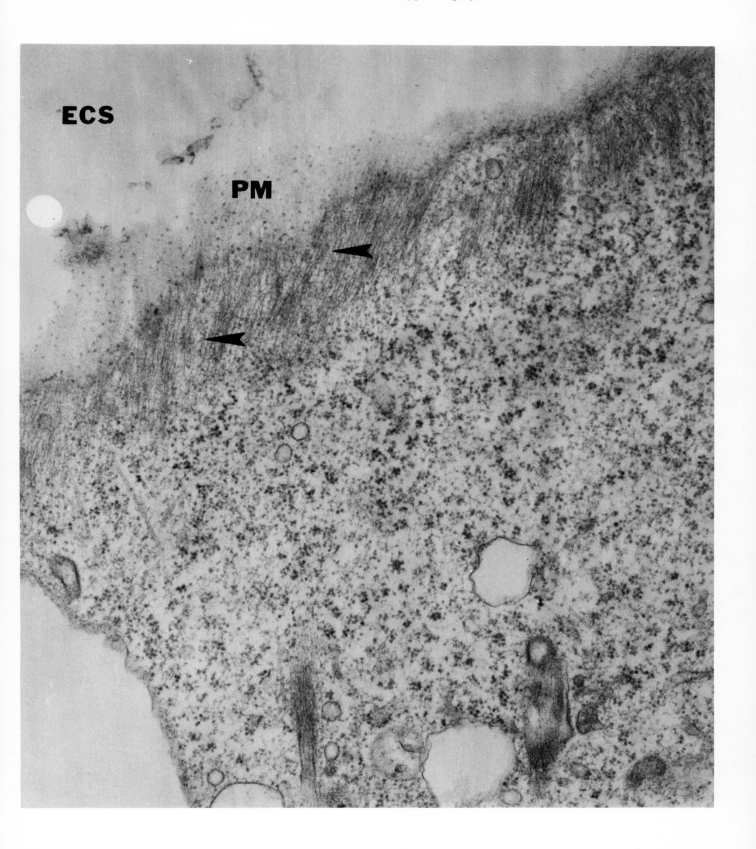

Figure 10. *The Z band substance (arrow) in this portion of a human ventricular cell has proliferated and extends an arm in either direction just under the sarcolemma of the myofiber. ECS = extracellular space. Z = Z band. (x 64,000).*

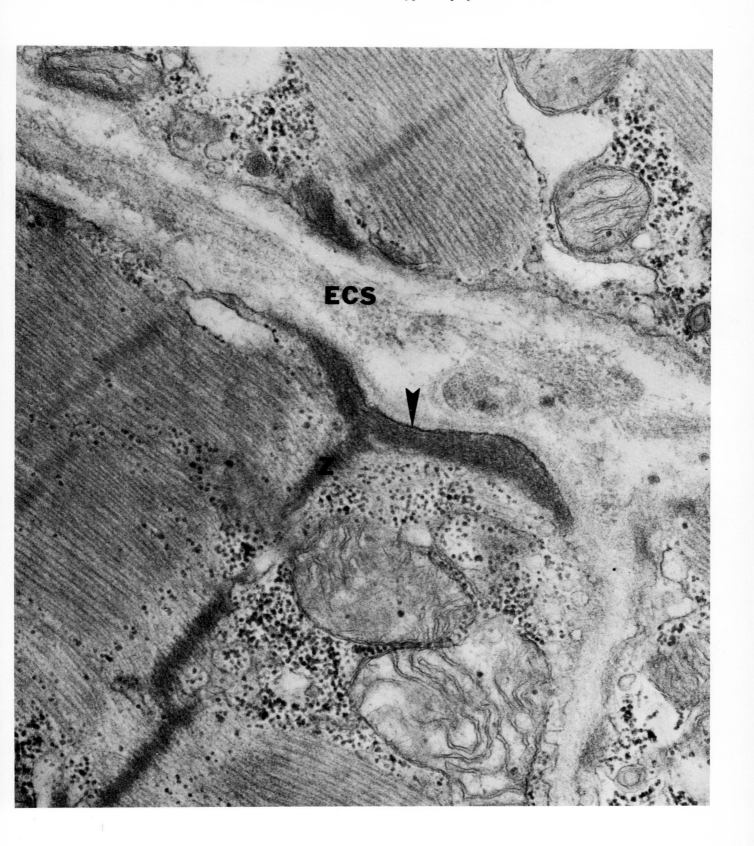

Figure 11. *Subsarcolemmal Z substance from adjacent Z bands has proliferated and joined to form an arch of Z substance under the cell membrane. Note that differentiated thin and thick sarcomeric myofilaments (arrows) are being laid down in register with the pre-existing sarcomeric components. (See text). Z = Z substance; ECS = extracellular space. (x 77,333).*

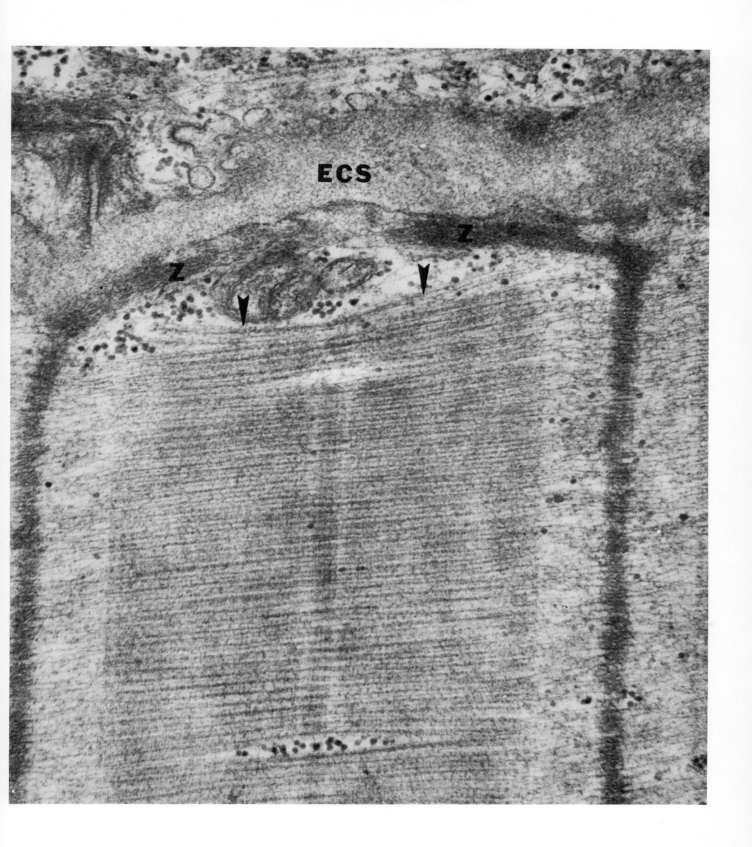

Figure 12a and b. *This shows the fine structure of a hypertrophied Z band (Z) deep within the cell. (x 123,515). The artist's sketch emphasizes the intricate patterning and consistent periodicity of the substructure. The Y-shaped insertion of the thin filament in the mass of accumulated Z substance is preserved, indicating that Z substance proliferation does not begin at the edge of the Z band and encroach upon thin filament organization, but starts in the center of the Z band and proceeds by pushing adjacent sarcomeres apart (see text).*

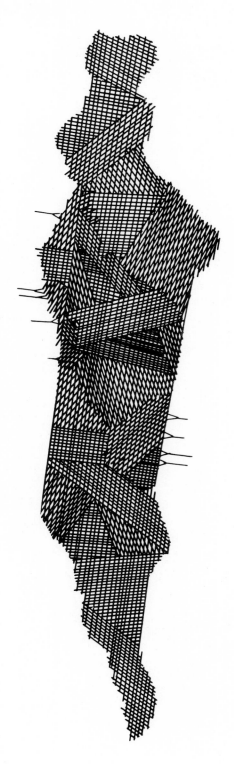

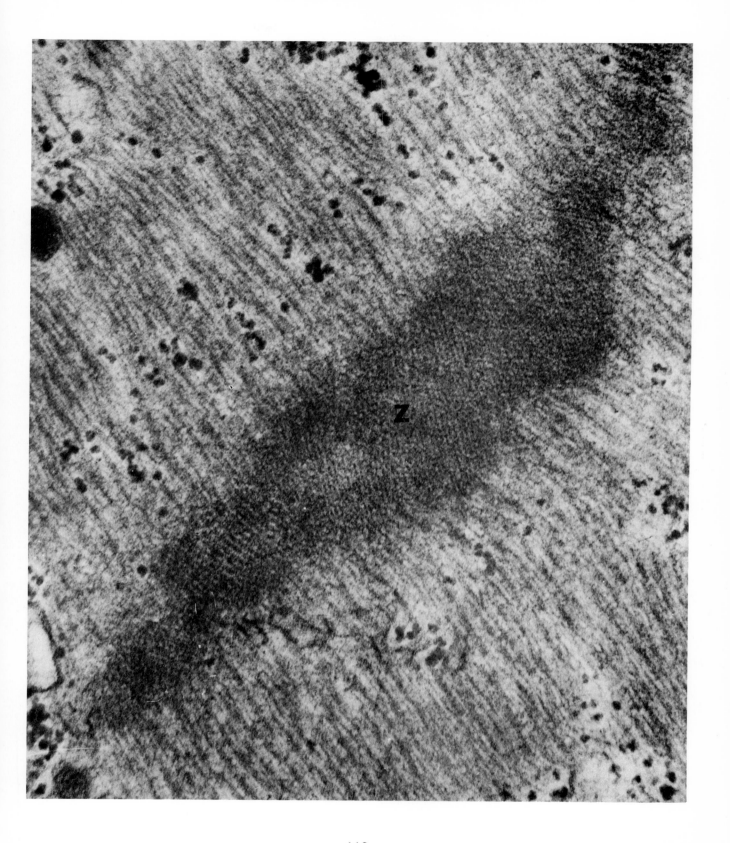

Figure 13a and b. *This electron micrograph shows the bilateral symmetry of the Z accumulation (Z). (x 103,477).*
The artist's sketch emphasizes the regular periodicity of the mass, which has a highly ordered substructure.

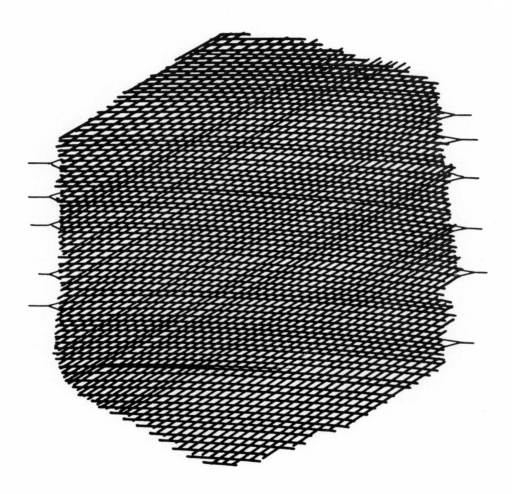

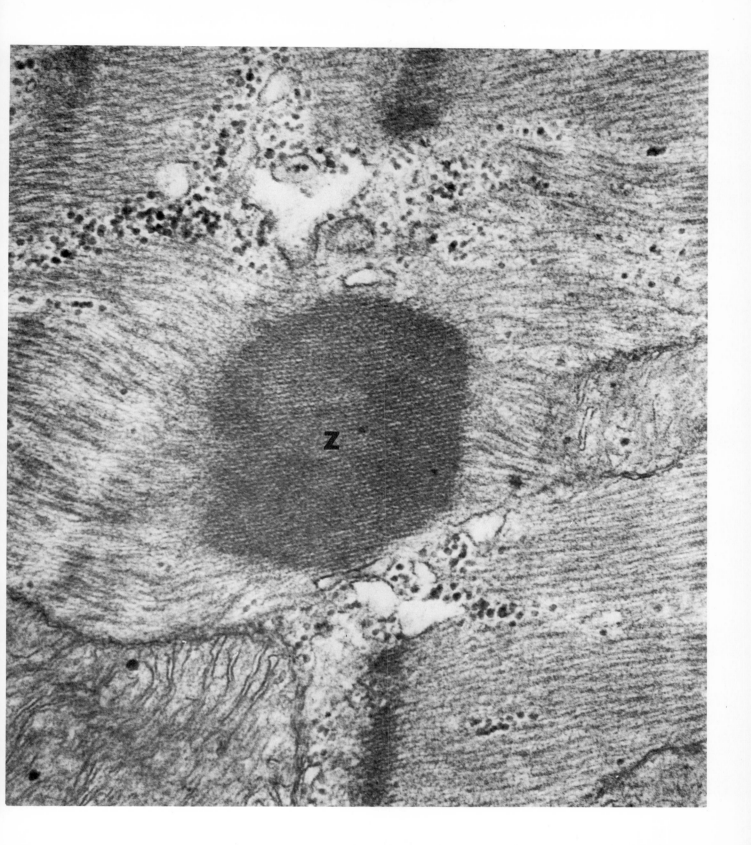

Figure 1.4. *This picture shows a maximally hypertrophied collection of Z substance (Z), which is almost the length of a sarcomere, (x 62,666).*

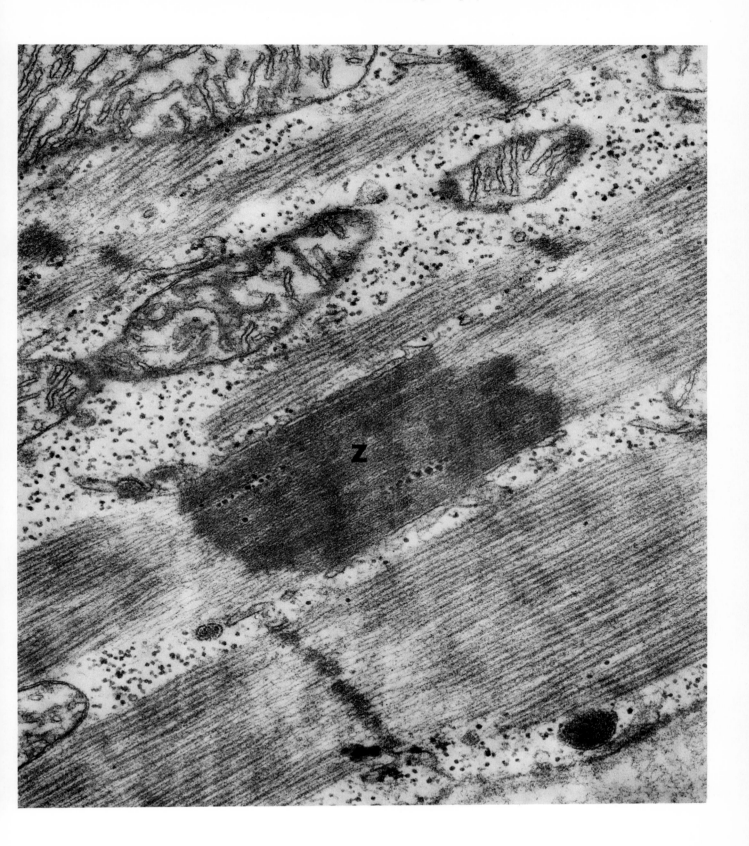

Figure 15. *After maximally hypertrophying, Z substance differentiates in the midportion into a homogenous group of filaments, the primary myofilaments (PM) (see text). These are further differentiated into sarcomeric thin and thick filaments to form a finished sarcomere. (x 69,333).*

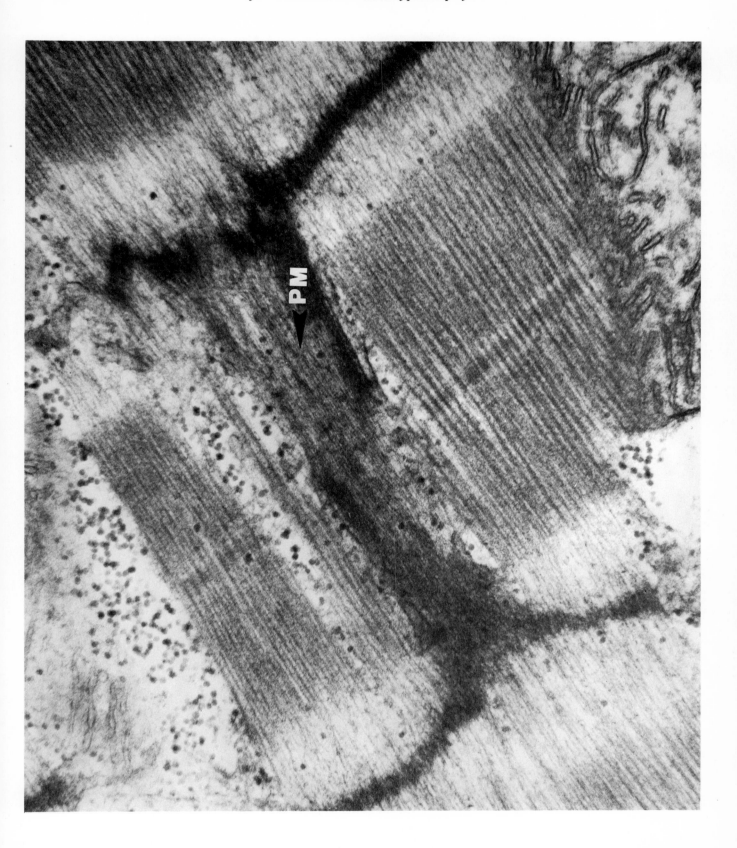

The same phenomenon, of an increase in Z substance with differentiation of Z material into primary myofilaments which in turn developed into thin and thick filaments was occurring at those areas of the intercalated disc where Z material is normally found in young and growing or adult hypertrophying cells.

Z substance apparently plays an important generative role in the production of new sarcomeric units in the cell (Figure 16). Polyribosomes are often seen aligned with myosin filaments in association with these developing and differentiating myofilaments, indicating that either the primary myofilaments may act as a substrate upon which the newly constructed myofilaments can be arranged in the proper order so that a new sarcomere is formed, or that primary myofilaments may actually be transformed or further differentiated into sarcomeric components. In this way, the adult cell, which has lost the capacity to divide, can still produce new sarcomeric units and thus add volume and contractile mass to the myofiber.

The second important cellular component to increase in number in the hypertrophied myofiber is the mitochondrion. The mitochondrion, (see Chapter IV) has its own genetic information and forms its whole system of inner cristae and many of its soluble components under the guidance of its own DNA. It does not depend, except for its outer membrane, on nuclear information. The mitochondrion grows to a critical size, its cristae increasing in number until its inner volume is filled with closely packed leaflets, and then divides by simple fission, and in so doing distributes its own DNA to each of the daughter units (See Chapter IV, Figures 2, 3, 4). Many examples of mitochondrial division are apparent in hypertrophied cells.

What role, if any, mitochondrial DNA plays in the production of new sarcomeres is not known. Mitochondrial and nuclear DNA are different molecules: one, for example, is a helix and the other a closed ring. It is possible that mitochondrial genetic information is not useful for extra-mitochondrial protein production. Mitochondria do contain ribosomes, however, and it is conceivable that they play some role in the production of new sarcomeric protein in the hypertrophying cell.

Causes of Congestive Heart Failure in the Hypertrophied Myocardium

The proteins produced in the new sarcomeres of the hypertrophied cell are probably, in essence, no different from that of the normal cell, although some investigators maintain that myosin isolated from failing myofibers has a diminished ATPase (4). Others have shown a diminished ability of sarcoplasmic reticulum to accumulate calcium in congestive heart failure (see Chapter V). Still others have suggested that a mitochondrial defect is the key deficiency in hypertrophy and congestive heart failure, but no one has demonstrated a deficiency of energy production *or* utilization in the failing myocardium (5). Unfortunately the cause of congestive failure at a cellular level continues to elude us. We still have no clue, in spite of growing insight into the mechanisms of myocardial hypertrophy, as to what makes such myocardium eventually decompensate.

Mechanism of Digitalis Action in the Myocardium

The exact mechanism of how digitalis produces an increased inotropism in cardiac tissue is still unknown (6). It is probably fair to say, however, that we are close to an answer. The number of cross bridge-active site linkages formed in the sarcomere is directly related to the amount of calcium presented to the myofilaments; as we discussed in Chapter III, the more calcium added to the sarcomere, the more of these linkages are made and the greater the resultant muscle systolic force generated. As we have also seen, the calcium that is presented to the area of the myofilaments is probably perimembrane calcium itself. It may be, however, calcium displaced from an internal releasing site by perimembrane calcium in the cell which is, in turn, delivered to the area of the myofilaments.

Langer advances the following theory (7, 8) about the action of digitalis in the myofiber: any increase in intracellular sodium facilitates the entry of calcium into the myofiber at the moment of depolarization. Digitalis retards the action of the sarcolemmal sodium pump (also called the membrane Na^+-K^+ ATPase) which ejects sodium from the cell, so that there is a build up of that cation in the digitalized myofiber. This increases the amount of calcium entering the cell at the moment of depolarization, which, Langer maintains, is the reason for the increment in systolic force induced by digitalis. From this, it would follow that the heart must be beating to be digitalized: unless there is entry of sodium into the cell at the moment of depolarization, compromise of the sodium pump will have only a small and delayed effect. Although there is a small resting flux of sodium across the cell membrane during diastole, the majority of the increase in intracellular sodium concentration is, of course, the consequence of depolarization (see Chapter II). Just as important in this respect is the fact that it is the calcium crossing the sarcolemma at the moment of depolarization which generates, directly or indirectly, systolic force in the cell.

Katz reminds us in a recent paper that calcium entry into the cell at the time of depolarization probably occurs primarily during the plateau of the action potential (9). He reasons, as Langer does, that digitalis augments the amount of calcium that enters the myofiber and suggests that those cells with the longest plateaus (and hence the longest action potentials) would be the cells most sensitive to digitalis action. There is indirect experimental evidence to support this proposition. Exact quantitation of the amount of calcium that crosses the cell during the action potential with and without digitalis is necessary to prove this, however, and at the moment we do not have this data.

An alternate mechanism of digitalis action is offered by Besch and Schwartz, who suggest that digitalis actually changes the configuration of the membrane Na^+, K^+—ATPase so that it binds calcium inside the sarcolemma, at the site where Na^+ is usually bound. Depolarization would result in the release of Ca^{++} so bound to the area of the myofilaments with resultant increased muscle inotropism (10).

Langer suggests that the ability of digitalis to poison the sodium pump may be the reason dilantin reverses digitalis intoxication; dilantin augments the activity of the sodium-potassium ATPase of the cell membrane. This also remains to be experimentally substantiated.

Figure 16. *This is a summary of the four principal steps in the evolution of a new sarcomeric unit from Z substance.*

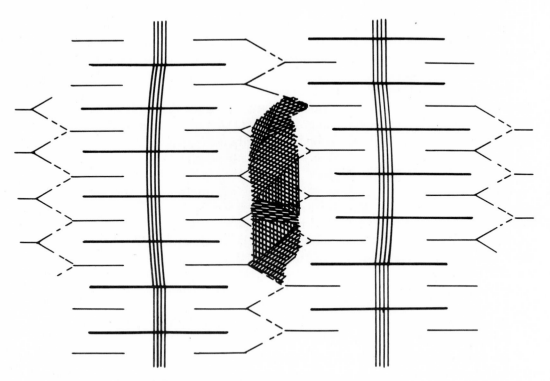

Stage I: Early hypertrophy of Z substance.

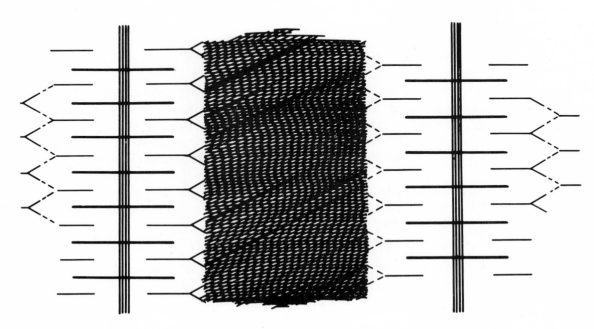

Stage II: Maximum hypertrophy of Z substance.

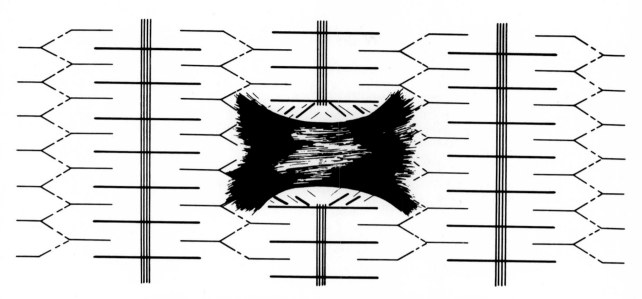

Stage III: Differentiation of Z substance into primary myofilaments.

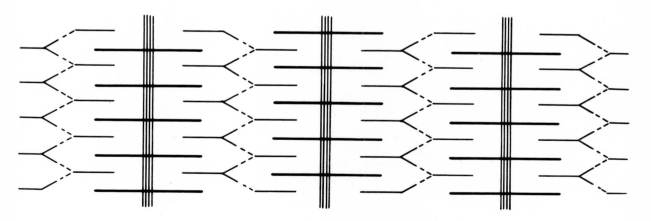

Stage IV: Production of a new, finished sarcomere.

Specific References

1. Legato, M. J.: Ultrastructural Characteristics of the Rat Ventricular Cell Grown in Tissue Culture, with Special Reference to Sarcomerogenesis. *J. Mol. Cell. Cardiol.*, 4:299, 1972.
2. Legato, M. J.: Sarcomerogenesis in Human Myocardium. *J. Mol. Cell. Cardiol.* 1:425, 1970.
3. Hagopian, M.: Derivation of the Z Line in the Embryonic Chick Heart. *J. Cell. Biol.*, 44:683, 1970.
4. Chandler, B. M., Sonnenblick, E. H., Spann, J. F. Jr., and Pool, P. E.: Association of Depressed Myofibrillar Adenosine Triphosphatase and Reduced Contractility in Experimental Heart Failure. *Circ. Res.*, 21:717, 1967.
5. Pool, P. E.: The Biochemical Basis of Heart Failure. *Hosp. Prac.*, 6:83, 1971.
6. Lee, K. S. and Klaus, W.: The Subcellular Basis for the Mechanism of Isotropic Action of Cardiac Glycosides. *Pharm. Rev.*, 23:193, 1971.
7. Langer, G. A.: The Mechanism of Action of Digitalis. *Hosp. Prac.*, 5:49, 1970.
8. Langer, G. A.: Effects of Digitalis on Myocardial Ionic Exchange. *Circ.*, 46:180, 1972.
9. Katz, A. M.: Increased Ca^{2+} Entry During the Plateau of the Action Potential: A Possible Mechanism of Cardiac Glycoside Action. *J. Mol. Cell. Cardiol.*, 4:87, 1972.
10. Besch, H. R., Jr. and Schwartz, A.: On a Mechanism of Action of Digitalis. *J. Mol. Cell. Cardiol.*, 1:195, 1970.

General References

Alpert, N. R. (Ed.): *Cardiac Hypertrophy.* Academic Press, New York, 1971.

CHAPTER VII

The Atrial, Purkinje and Ventricular Cell

Functionally and morphologically, there are four types of cells in the heart. The working cells of the atria and ventricles, although they differ from one another, have the same primary role: to perform contractile work. These, together with the specialized conducting and pacemaking cell, the Purkinje fiber (modifications of which can be found in both atrial and ventricular tissue), make up the majority of the myocardial population. There are also specialized groups of cells in the sinus and atrio-ventricular nodes: these are called P, or pale cells because of their appearance and were described by Thomas James (1, 2). Their actual function is not known and their ultrastructure will not be reviewed in detail here.

Interestingly, the interior morphology of these four cell groups is not very dissimilar. They all have the same basic set of organelles. Functionally, though, they are very disparate. Their essential differences lie in their electrical properties. Each, for example, generates a unique and characteristic action potential. They conduct impulses at different speeds and have different measured values for membrane capacitance and resistance (Table I). These variations are the consequence to some extent of cell geometry, but primarily are due to different membrane characteristics—not only the nature and extent of the derivatives of the cell membrane in the myofiber (the transverse tubular system and the system of intercellular linkages) but also, more fundamentally, to differences in membrane molecular architecture and composition. Only the latter can explain the differences in ionic permeability characteristics which are responsible for the variation in action potential between these cell groups and whether or not they have pacemaking ability. Indeed, as a recent thoughtful study by Wallace's group has emphasized, membrane permeability characteristics differ between cell types in subtle and complex ways we do not fully understand or appreciate at the present time (3).

It should be emphasized that there are no sharp distinctions between cells which are primarily conducting or pacing and those which perform contractile work either anatomically or functionally. There are, rather, so called transitional cells at the boundaries between specialized conducting or pacing and ordinary working cells which have morphologic characteristics of both groups. Whether these are the same cells which are in the well demonstrated *electrophysiologic* or *functional* transition zone between Purkinje fibers and the working myocardium is not demonstrated, but it is reasonable to suspect that this might be the case.

The Atrial Cell

The working atrial cell is an oval or elliptical myofiber about 6-8μ wide and 20-30μ long which, in contrast to its counterpart in the ventricle, does not usually

TABLE 1
RELATIONSHIP OF ULTRASTRUCTURAL FEATURES OF PURKINJE AND VENTRICULAR FIBERS TO ELECTRICAL CONSTANTS AND CONDUCTION VELOCITY IN THE TISSUE

	PURKINJE CELL	VENTRICULAR CELL	RELATED ULTRASTRUCTURAL DETAILS
CONDUCTION VELOCITY = $\dfrac{K \times radius\ of\ cell}{C_m \times R_m}$	4 Meters/sec	1 Meter/sec	
Cell diameter	35-40 microns	10-15 microns	
Membrane capacitance (C_m)	12.8 microfara-days/cm^2	0.81 microfara-days/cm^2	Purkinje cell has sarcolemmal evaginations and much more entensive intercalated disc than the ventricular cell.
Membrane resistance (Rm)	1220-1700 ohms/cm^2	9100 ohms/cm^2	Ventricular cells have an extensive T system and a much less extensive intercalated disc; either may be related to higher Rm in ventricular cells.

branch (Figures 1 a, b, and c, 2, 3). Atrial cells are juxtaposed in a rather unique way; their system of intercellular connections is very different from that of ventricular tissue. They are placed close together in ribbons of 2-3 cells, so that they are often not more than 200-300 Å apart along the entire extent of their lateral borders. The sarcolemmae of both cells pursue an exactly parallel, undulating course, the substance of their perimembranes intermingling. Intermittently, the plasma membranes of the sarcolemma join in specialized linkages to form either isolated desmosomal connections or a sequence of desmosomal and nexal junctions which constitute a short intercalated disc, oriented parallel to the long axis of the cell. Rarely, the specialized portion of the disc is oriented perpendicularly to the long axis of the cell, but this is the exception and not the rule in atrial tissue. This arrangement of intercellular junctions allows for impulse transmission between atrial cells in both a side-to-side as well as end-to-end direction. The multiplicity and diversity of intercellular linkages may explain the persistence of abnormal rhythms in atrial tissue, where cells have multiple points which allow impulse re-entry and where temporal differences in refractoriness can occur. Moreover, bundles of atrial cells are separated by wide areas of collagen, in which are embedded capillaries and fibroblasts; this alternation of islands of closely packed myofibers separated by broad areas of interstitial space may explain the persistence of chronic arrhythmias like atrial fibrillation for many years; the atria may be envisioned in such a circumstance as a collection of isolated areas of re-entering electrical activity separated by and insulated from one another by relatively broad lakes of connective tissue. It also may explain the propensity of atria afflicted by diseases which increase the amount of connective tissue between cell groups, such as rheumatic and advanced arteriosclerotic heart disease, to fibrillate. This does not occur in ventricular tissue, where tissue architecture is very different; cells branch and are connected to one another almost exclusively via end-to-end linkages. They have only rare side-to-side connections and the amount of collagen in the interstitial compartment is really very small. The ratio of myofibers to interstitial space is much higher in ventricular tissue than in the atrial myocardium; the ventricle is a thick walled, strongly contracting chamber which must propel blood against considerable resistance. The atria, in contrast, are required to generate much less contractile force except at the end of diastole; it performs the dual function of impulse transmission and passive reception of blood from the greater and lesser circulations. It requires therefore a much lower proportion of contractile elements and indeed, this is the case.

The atrial cell, with an occasional exception, has no transverse tubular system. It has an abundance of peripheral coupling sites, however, and a modification of the sarcoplasmic reticular network at the Z band which is called a "dense coated vesicle"—the SR tubule expands into a round globular sac, often comes into apposition with a similar modification of the sarcoplasmic reticulum from the adjacent sarcomere (Figure 4). The two vesicles are separated by a thin central tubule which lies over the Z band and the resultant configuration is, anatomically at least, analogous to the triads and diads of the ventricular cell (Figure 2). Whether the thin, central tubule of the configuration is open to the extracellular space is unknown. It is not labelled by the electron dense substances used to mark the extracellular space, such as peroxidase or sodium antimonate, but this may be due to its very small diameter, which will not allow unimpeded diffusion of substances from the extracellular compartment at the surface of the cell into the narrow tubular lumen. The whole question of whether or not an anatomic substrate exists to provide for the internal release of calcium at multiple levels of the myofiber in response to excitation in the atrial, or for that matter, in the ventricular cell is unsettled (See Chapters 2 and 5).

The atrial myofiber has an interesting organelle not found in ventricular or Purkinje fibers called the "specific granule" (Figures 1, 2, 3, and 5). These are membrane-limited very electron dense spheres which are most abundant at the nuclear poles but which are also found between myofibrils in the body of the cell and in the subsarcolemmal area (Figure 3). Their function is unknown; they are not Periodic Acid Shift (PAS) positive, indicating that they are not carbohydrate, do not contain lipid, and are probably primarily composed of protein (5). Although there is some evidence to suggest that their number is lessened in the reserpinized animal (6), it is not demonstrated that they contain catecholamines as do the residual bodies of the ventricular cell (5). They are more abundant in animals with more rapid heart rates (4), but they bear no constant relationship to the superficial membrane systems of the cell and cannot, on an anatomic basis, at least, be implicated in excitation—contraction coupling in the cell.

The Purkinje Cell

The specialized conducting tissue of the heart is composed of very broad (sometimes as much as 50 μ in diameter) cells (Figures 6 a and b) which have the most extensively developed intercalated discs in the heart (Figure 7). There is a wide

Figure 1a. *This is a portion of three atrial cells. Note the serpentine course of their parallel sarcolemmae which fuse (arrows) in a series of specialized linkages. (x 9,333).*

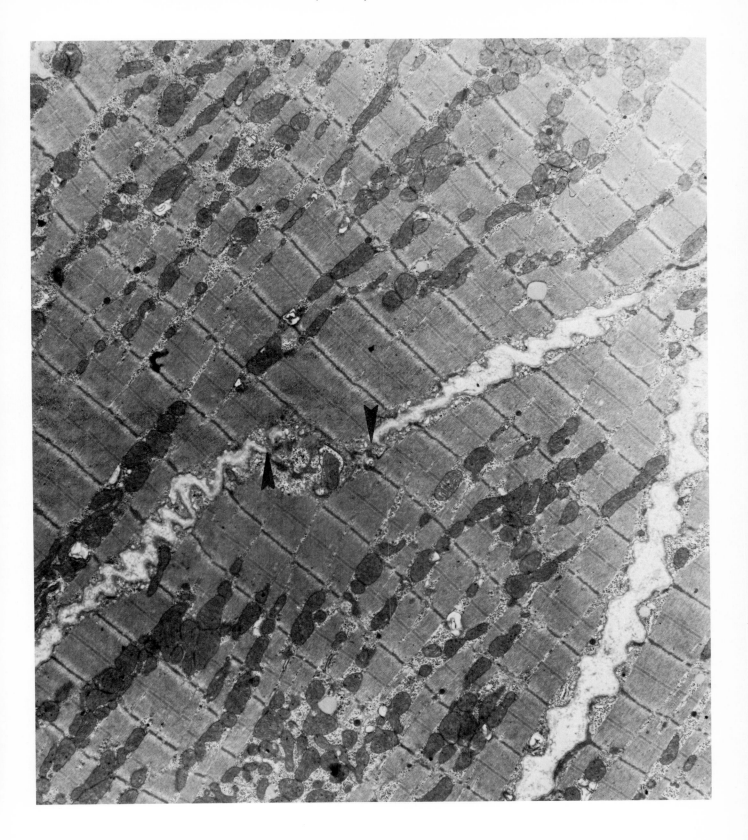

Figure 1b. This micrograph shows a rare orientation of the intercalated disc (arrows) for atrial tissue; it is perpendicular to the long axis of the cell. AG = atrial granules. (x 9,333).

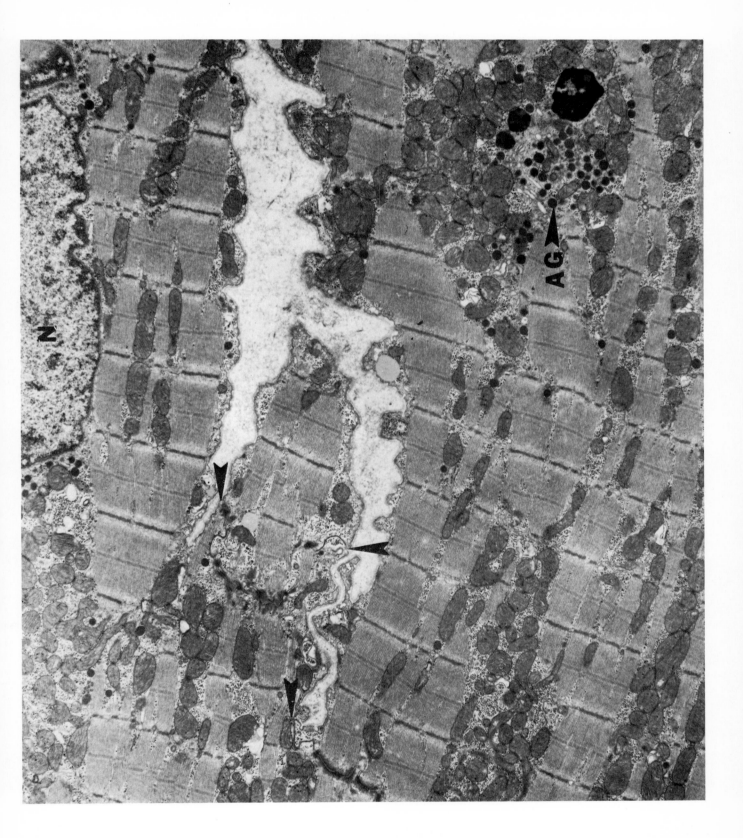

Figure 1c. *This is a sketch of two adjacent atrial cells which illustrates the primary features of these myofibers. Note the parallel undulating course of adjacent sarcolemmae which terminates in a series of specialized intercellular connections. (One sarcomere in this sketch represents 10-12 sarcomeres in the actual cell.).*

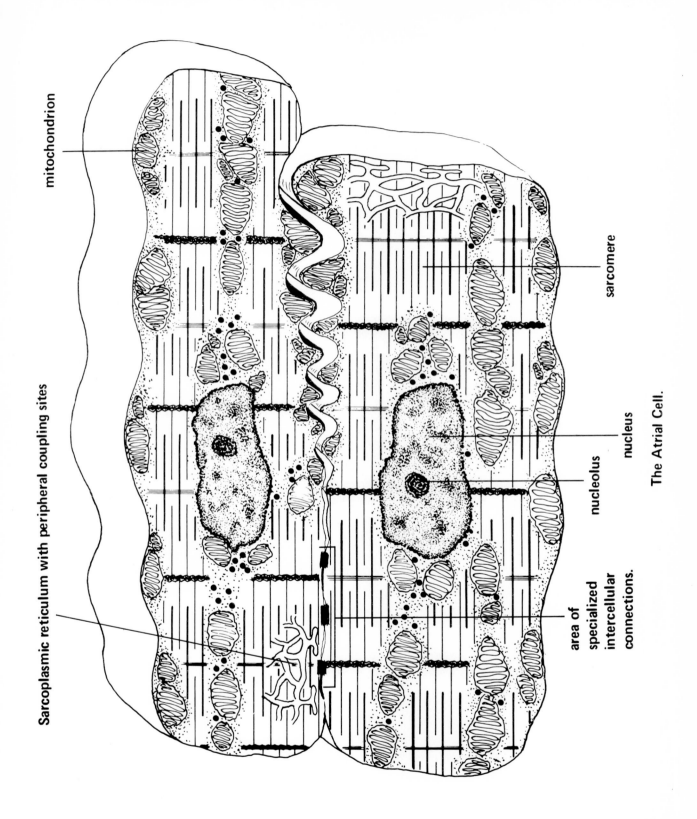

mitochondrion

Sarcoplasmic reticulum with peripheral coupling sites

sarcomere

nucleus

nucleolus

The Atrial Cell.

area of specialized intercellular connections.

Figure 2. *This high power view of portions of two adjacent atrial cells shows the abundance of specialized connections (arrows) which lie parallel to the long axis of the cell. N = nucleus. (x 12,000).*

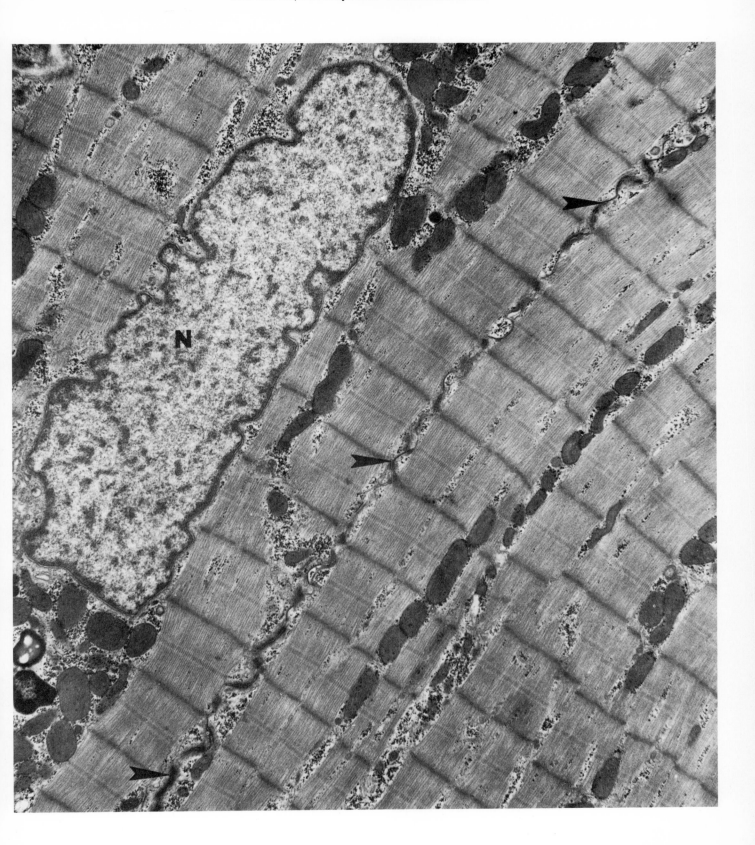

Figure 3. *This fragment of atrial tissue shows the area of the nuclear pole which contains mitochondria (M), glycogen and atrial granules (AG) as well as a prominent golgi apparatus (GA). N = nucleus. ECS = extracellular space. C = capillary. (x 10,686).*

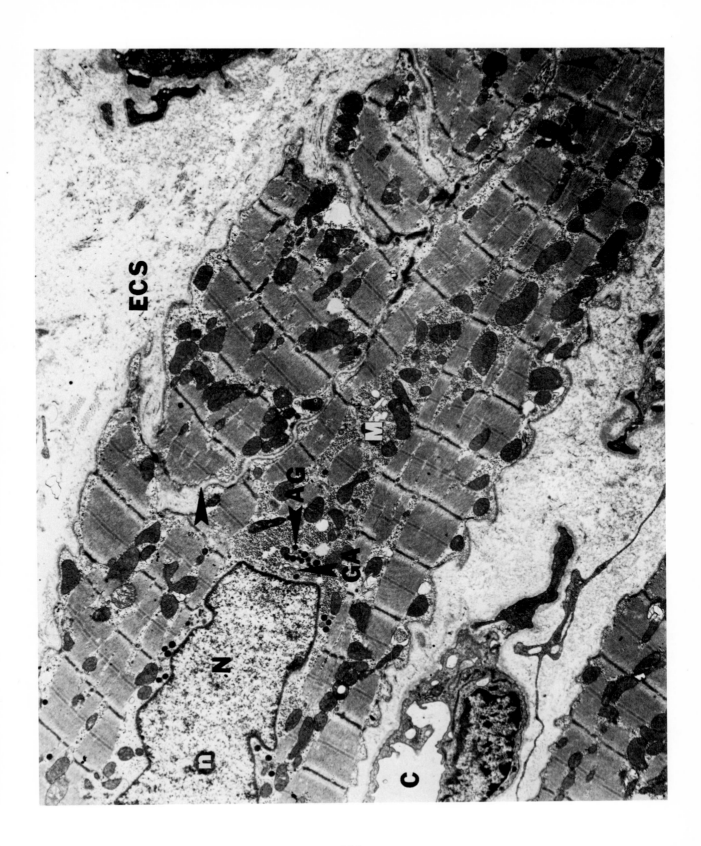

Figure 4. *This portion of an atrial cell shows a possible anatomic substrate for excitation-contraction coupling in the atrial cell, which is without a transverse tubular system. Two dense coated vesicles parenthesize a narrow central tubule in a triadic configuration (circle). (x 29,333).*

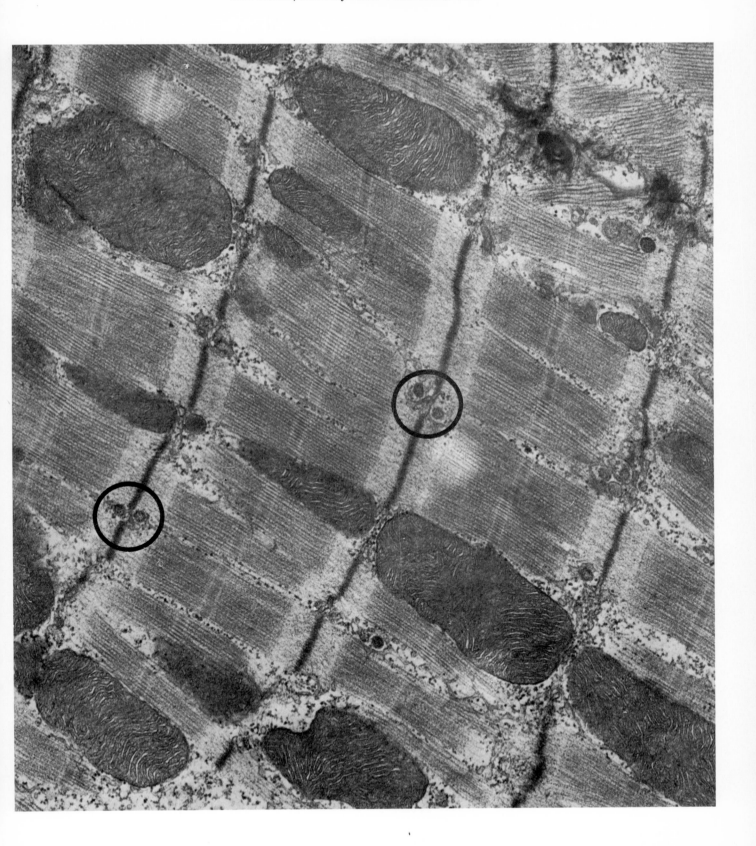

Figure 5. *This is a high power view of atrial granules (arrows) showing their spherical contour and the granular nature of the material in their interior. (x 48,856).*

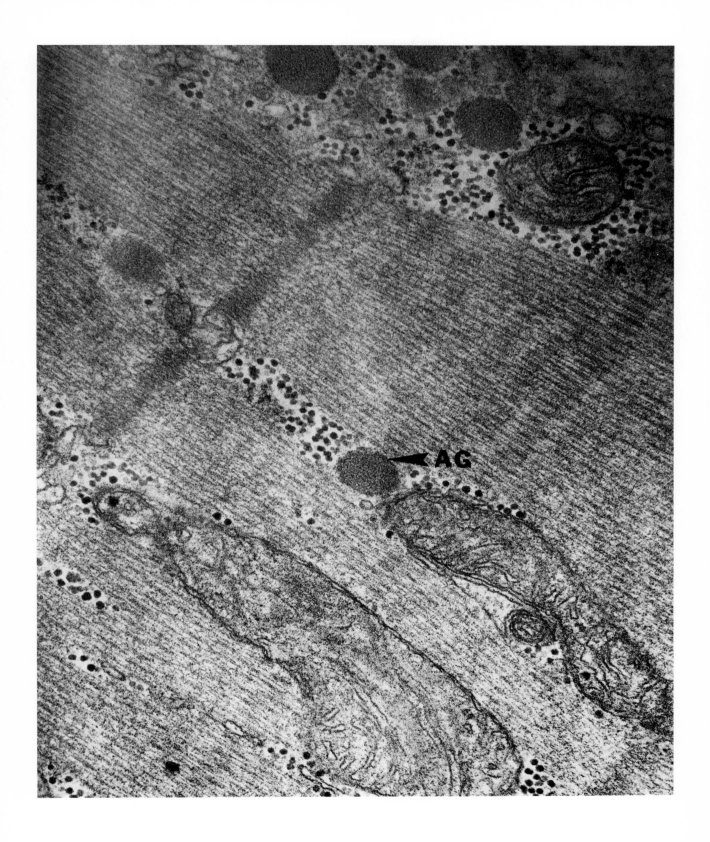

Figure 6a. *This is a portion of a Purkinje cell in the ventricular myocardium. It shows large pools of glycogen and mitochondria characteristic of these cells. Note that some are subsarcolemmal. N = nucleus. ECS = extracellular space. GP = glycogen pool. Myofibrils run in clusters parallel to the long axis of the cell but do not fill the entire cell substance as they do in Figure 8. (x 7,052).*

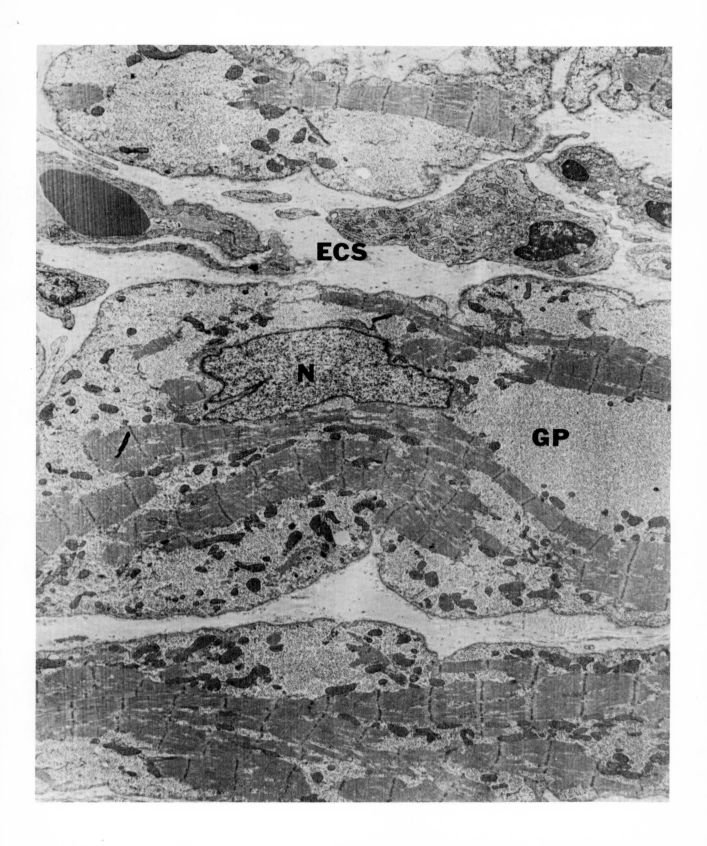

Figure 6b. *This sketch of the Purkinje cell shows the characteristic features of the unit. There is no transverse tubular system, but instead an abundance of peripheral coupling sites (PCS) (an approximation of the lateral sacs of the sarcoplasmic reticulum to the sarcolemma or to the unspecialized portion of the intercalated disc). Mitochondria filled glycogen pools are located in both subsarcolemmal and deeply intracellular positions. The intercalated disc (ID) has an abundant surface area with many specialized portions, both desmosomes (D) and nexuses (N). Note that the sarcomere is not in scale with the rest of the cell. This is in order to show detail: one sarcomere in this sketch represents approximately 10-15 sarcomeres.*

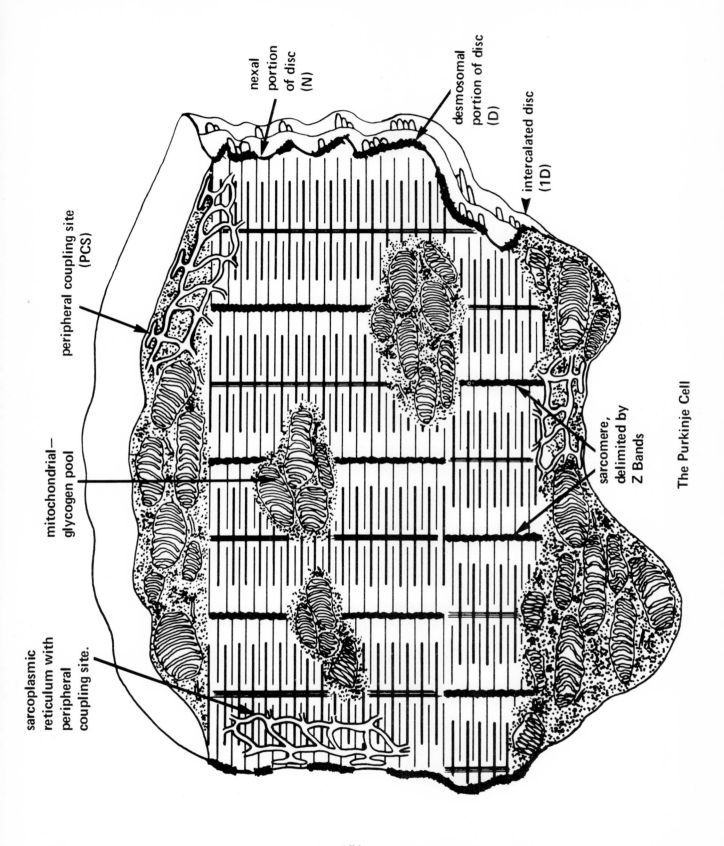

nexal portion of disc (N)

desmosomal portion of disc (D)

intercalated disc (1D)

peripheral coupling site (PCS)

mitochondrial— glycogen pool

sarcoplasmic reticulum with peripheral coupling site.

sarcomere, delimited by Z Bands

The Purkinje Cell

Figure 7. *This is an intercalated disc joining two Purkinje cells. Note its enormous surface area and the fact that along almost all of its extent are specialized linkages, both desmosomal (D) and nexal (N). (x 128,710).*

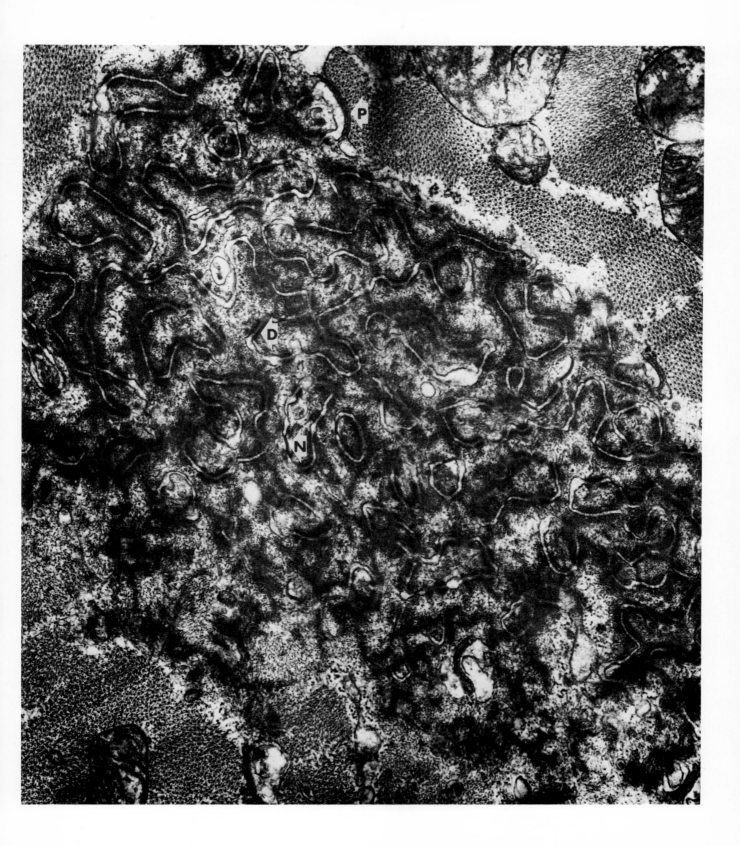

spectrum of intracellular organization: contrary to what is often written as characteristic of this type of myofiber, many Purkinje cells are packed with myofibrils and, except for the fact that they lack any vestige of a transverse tubular system, are indistinguishable from ordinary working ventricular cells (Figure 8). Often, however, they have large pools of intra-cellular glycogen (Figure 6). These may be deep within the cell or they may appear under the sarcolemma as large outpocketings of the cell membrane which enclose glycogen and mitochondria suspended in myofilament-free sarcoplasm (Figures 9, 10, 11). Weidmann has estimated that Purkinje cell internal resistance is 1/3 that of the ventricular myofiber (7). The large glycogen pools which are interspersed between myofibrils may be the reason for this; their resistance to the passage of current may be virtually negligible in contrast to the resistance offered by the close packed array of sarcomeric myofilaments which fill the whole substance of the ventricular cell.

The system of intercellular connections between Purkinje cells is remarkable for the extent of the intercalated disc and as a result, the extraordinarily high number of specialized linkages between cells (Figures 7, 12, 13). The fact that membrane capacitance in the Purkinje cell is twelve times that of the ventricular cell (8) (Table I), is probably related to the tremendous membrane surface area included in the extensive discs that join these myofibers. To a lesser extent, this may also be contributed to by the evaginations of the sarcolemma which enclose the submembranous glycogen pools characteristic of Purkinje cells. In some areas, the cells are arranged in an almost mosaic like pattern; they touch a neighboring cell on virtually all sides, and the widest gap that separates the myofibers in this part of the tissue is only 200Å-300Å wide (Figures 12, 13). At many points, the cell borders are fused in specialized junctions, primarily desmosomes. There is little question that the Purkinje cells have the most abundant specialized intercellular connections.

The rapid speed of conduction which is such a fundamental property of this tissue may be related to either the high number of specialized intercellular connections (the nexus and/or the desmosomes), the wide diameter of the cell, or to both. Conduction velocity is directly proportional to the cell radius and inversely proportional to membrane capacitance and resistance. The high capacitance value of the Purkinje cell is balanced by its very low membrane resistance (Rm) (1/3 that of the ventricular cell); the latter is probably the consequence of its extensive intercalated disc, which, as Weidmann so convincingly demonstrated, is a low resistance junction between cells (9). The relatively low Rm of the Purkinje cell may also be due to the absence of a transverse tubular system in these myofibers—a subcellular system which in contrast to Purkinje cells, is well developed in the ventricular myofiber.

Although the Purkinje tissue that has been best studied has been taken from the ventricles, Berger, who has done extensive and careful work on atrial cell ultrastructure, described a population of cells in the subendocardial layer of the rat atrium which has many of the characteristics of ventricular Purkinje tissue; they have a population of mitochondria with long, tapering tails said to be characteristics of Purkinje cells, they have areas of cytoplasm which are relatively clear, and they do not have the entire spectrum of granules which are characteristic of atrial working cells (Figure 14) (10). Although the electrophysiologic identification of such cells as pacemaking and rapidly conducting myofibers is lacking at the present time, it is likely that they are the Purkinje cells of the atrial myocardium.

The Ventricular Cell

The ordinary working ventricular myocardium is an aggregate of broad sheets of long $(30\text{-}40\mu)$ and narrow $(8\text{-}12\mu)$ cells, which branch frequently and are connected end-to-end through intercalated discs whose specialized portions are arranged perpendicularly to the long axes of the cells (Figures 15 a and b). The space between cells is uniform and wider than the space between either atrial or Purkinje myofibers, so that perimembranes of adjacent cells in general do not intermingle. The interior of the cell is, except in the perinuclear area, packed with orderly rows of myofibrils. Mitochondria are very abundant, perhaps more so than in any other type of cell in the heart. Glycogen is present, but is distributed primarily around mitochondria and does not exist in the large pools which interrupt myofibrillar organization in the Purkinje cell.

There is a well developed transverse tubular system; it is so abundant that a triadic or diadic unit exists for every sarcomere in the myofiber.

There are two types of electron dense organelles in the ventricular cell, the so-called residual bodies, which are high in catecholamine content, and lipofuscin bodies which are essentially aggregates of lipid; their number increases with the age of the cell, but their exact function is unknown (Figure 15A). In summary then, the morphology of the three principal groups of myocardial cells is as disparate as their functional characteristics. Many of the functional differences between cell types can be related to differences in their morphology. These differences, which are summarized in Table 2, are especially related to differences in their electrical properties (Table 1).

A better understanding of the role of subcellular systems in the myofiber and of the anatomic features characteristic of the major cell types in the myocardium cannot help but produce better insight into how the normal cell works to maintain myocardial function. This, in turn will allow us to pinpoint much more exactly the things that go wrong in the diseased and failing heart, and will, hopefully, immeasurably improve our therapeutic acumen.

Figure 8. *This micrograph illustrates that not all Purkinje cells contain prominent glycogen pools, but are filled with myofibrils. The only thing distinguishing such myofibers from ventricular cells is the absence of a transverse tubular system. Portions of five Purkinje cells are represented in this field. (They are numbered 1 through 5). (x 14,450).*

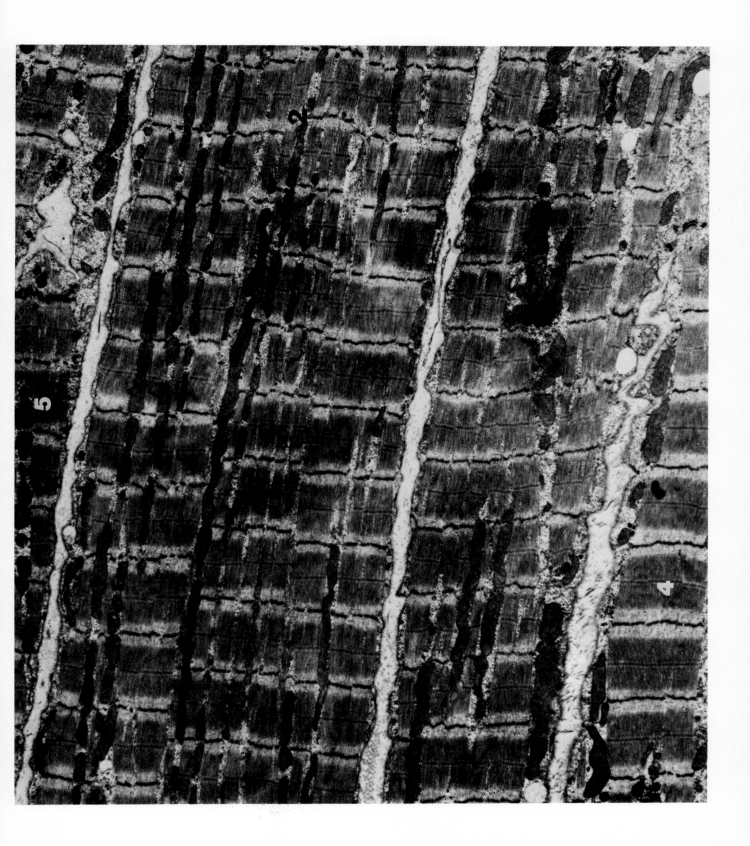

Figure 9. *Note the undulating course of the intercalated disc (arrows) that joins Purkinje cells. Contrast to arrangement of the intercellular connections between atrial (see Figures 1-3) and ventricular (see Figure 15a) cells. N = nucleus. White n = nucleolus. GP = glycogen pool. (x 5,133).*

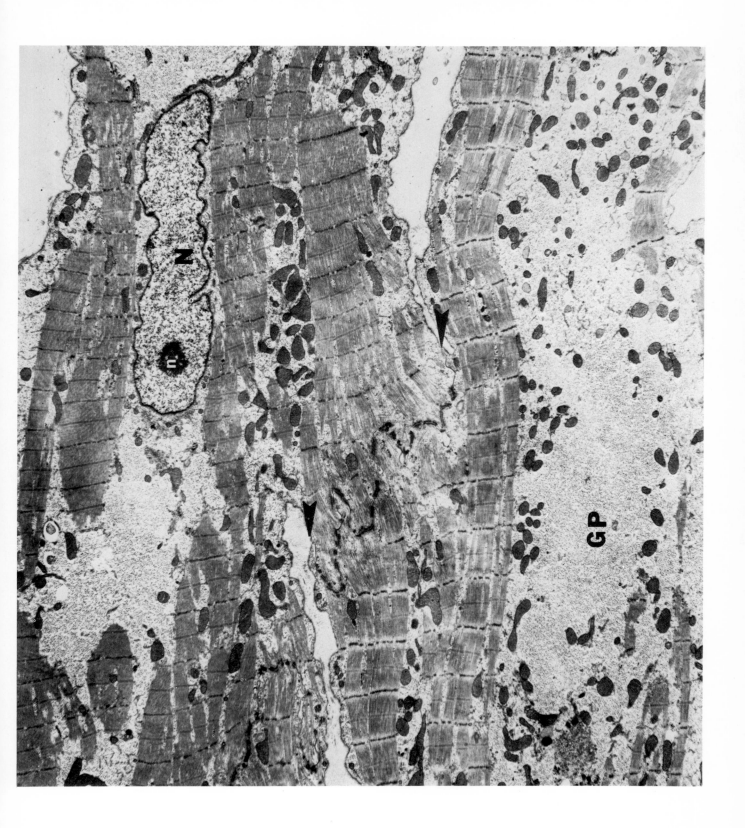

Figure 10. *This is a high power view of subsarcolemmal glycogen pools (GP) in a Purkinje cell. (x 7,200).*

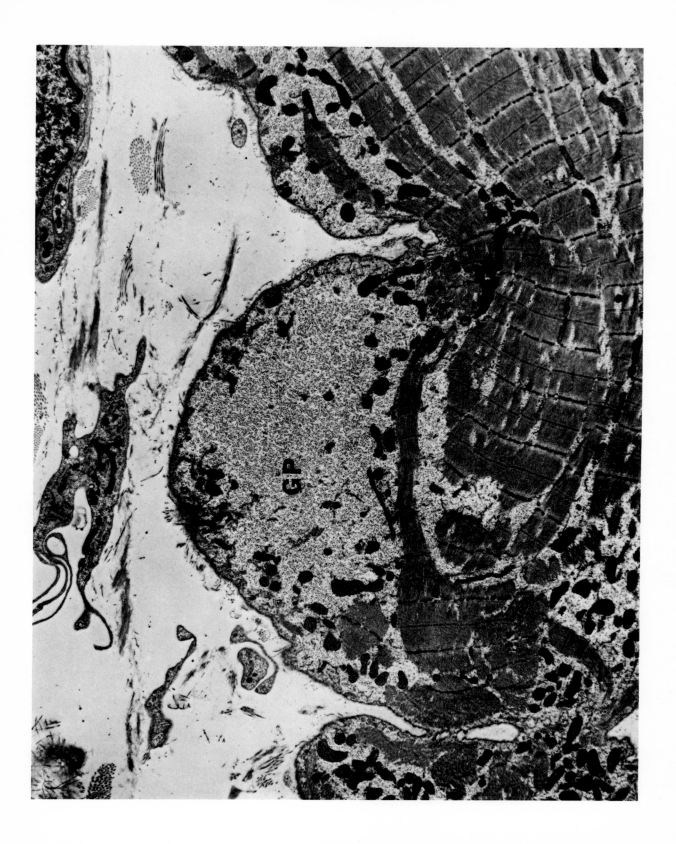

Figure 11. *Note the single myofibril (arrow) that separates the sarcolemma from the peripherally located glycogen pools (GP) in this Purkinje fiber. (x 8,160).*

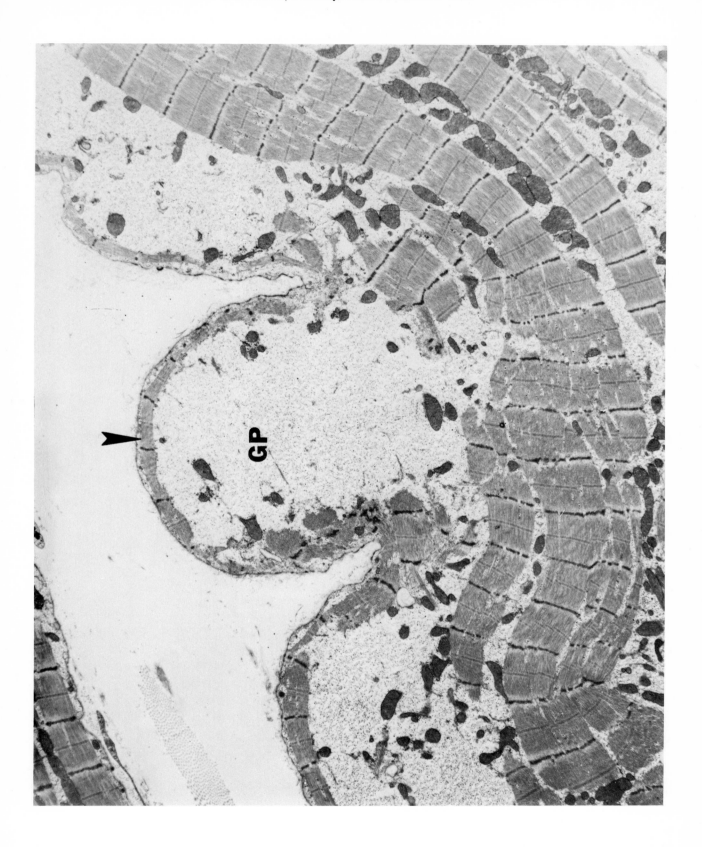

Figure 12. *Often Purkinje cells are arranged in an almost mosiac-like pattern; they are closely approximated to one another over most of their surfaces, and nexal and desmosomal linkages are placed all along the course of adjacent sarcolemma. Note the serpentine course the adjacent membranes of these two Purkinje cells follow from the upper right to lower left hand corner of the micrograph. N = nexus. D = desmosome. (x 28,387).*

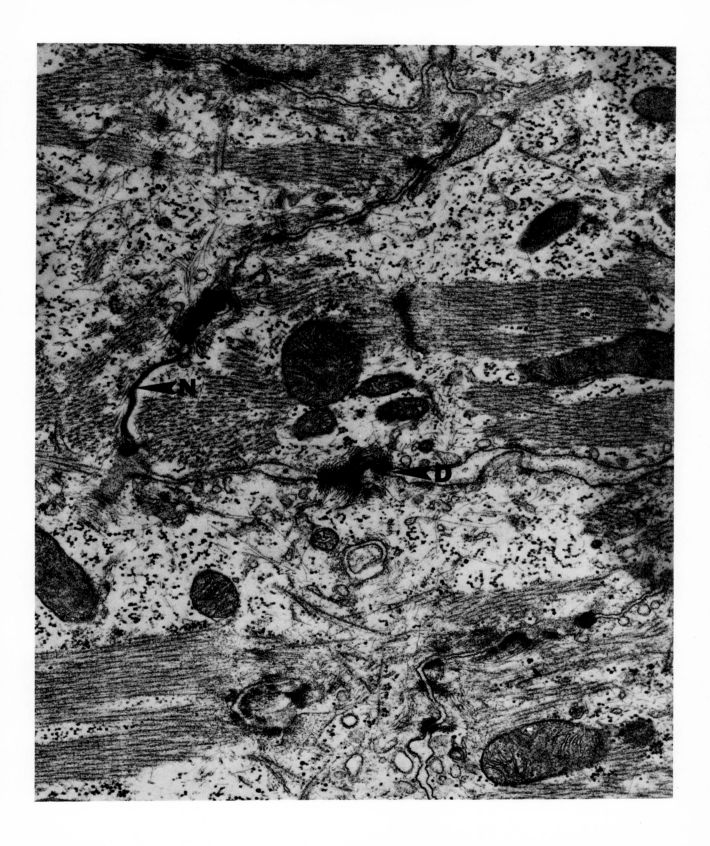

Figure 13. *Some of the longest nexal connections (N) in the heart are found joining Purkinje cells. (x 33,894).*

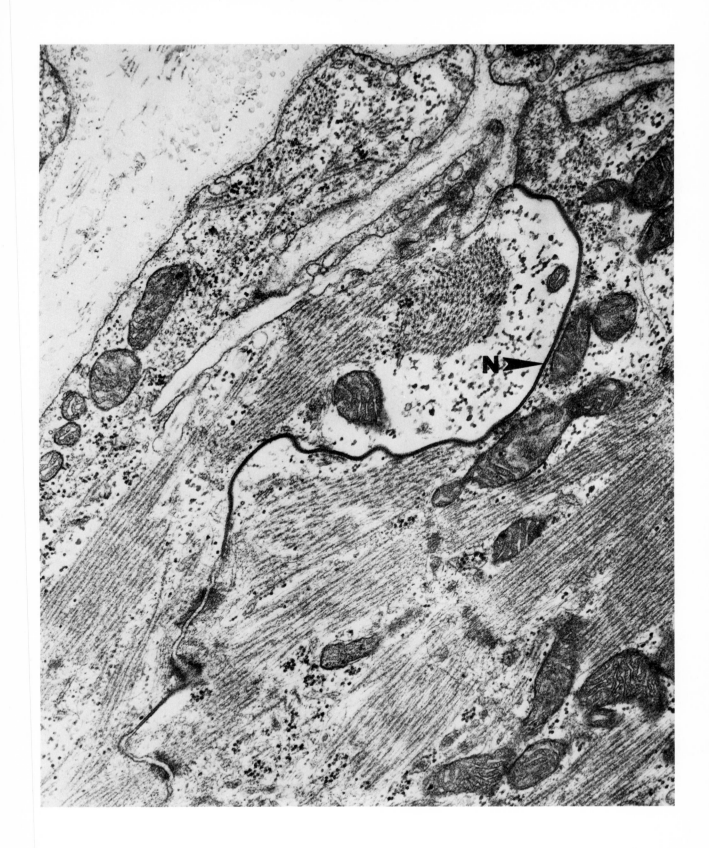

Figure 14. *This is a portion of a human atrial cell which shows many of the ultrastructural characteristics of Purkinje myofibers: note the large glycogen pool (arrows) filled with mitochondria (M). N = nucleus. n = nucleolus. (x 11,547).*

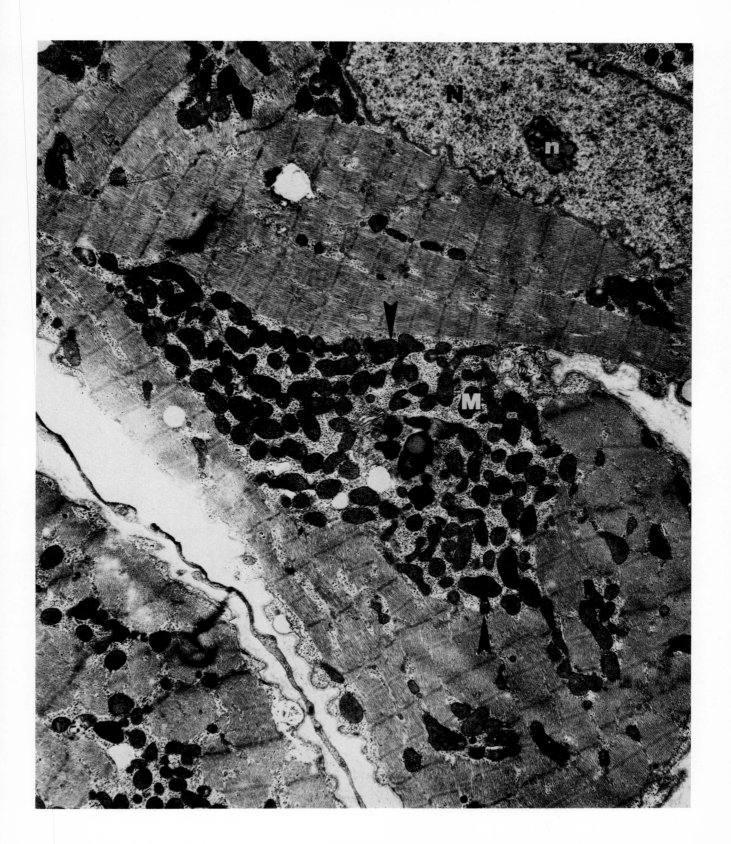

Figure 15a. *This micrograph shows portions of 4 working ventricular cells. Notice the long, narrow dimension of these cells, the presence of triadic and diadic units (circles) and the stepwise course of the intercalated disc (ID). N = nucleus. (x 7,000).*

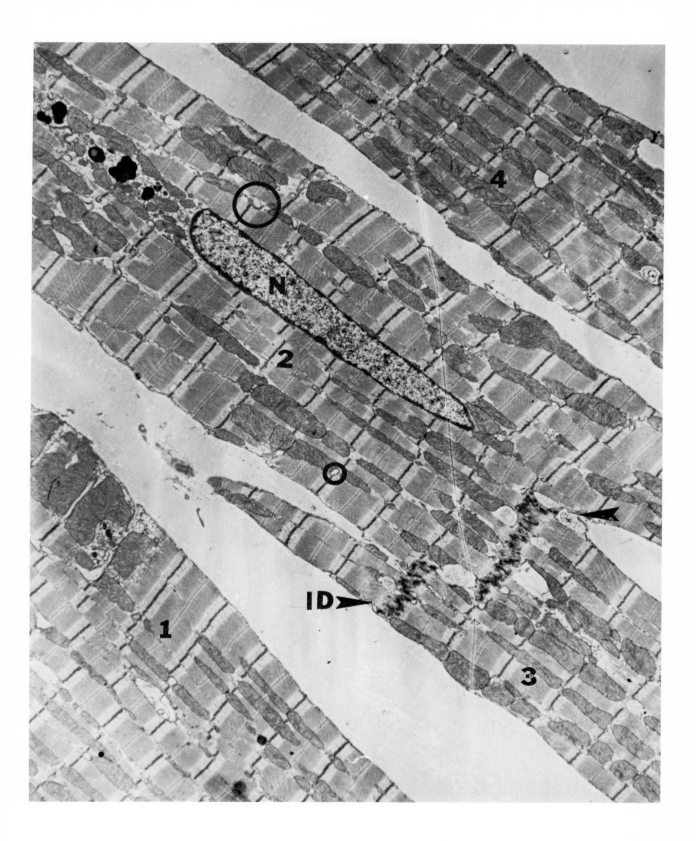

Figure 15b. *This sketch of the ventricular cell shows the ultrastructural characteristics of this population of cells in the heart. Note the origin of the transverse tubular system (TT) in the sarcolemma, and the relationship to it of the sarcoplasmic reticulum (SR). Both diadic (D) and triadic (T) units are present (M = mitochondria, S = sarcomere). Note the stepwise course of the intercalated disc in this cell population (ID); contrast to Figures 1b and 6b. Again, one sarcomere in this sketch represents 10-12 sarcomeres.*

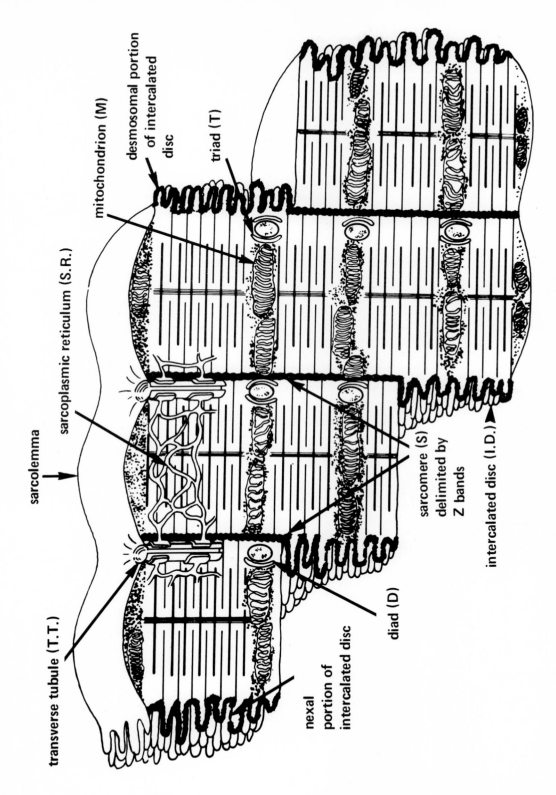

desmosomal portion of intercalated disc

mitochondrion (M)

triad (T)

sarcoplasmic reticulum (S.R.)

sarcolemma

transverse tubule (T.T.)

nexal portion of intercalated disc

diad (D)

sarcomere (S) delimited by Z bands

intercalated disc (I.D.)

The ordinary working ventricular cell

TABLE 2.
COMPARISON OF ULTRASTRUCTURAL FEATURES OF ATRIAL, VENTRICULAR AND PURKINJE CELLS: SUMMARY

	ATRIAL	VENTRICULAR	PURKINJE
DIMENSION AND SHAPE	elliptical (6-8μ wide x 20μ long)	narrow (15-20μ wide) and long (100μ); frequent branching	Broad (35-40μ in diameter)
CELL CONTENTS: Myofibrils	fundamentally identical organization in long parallel rows		
Mitochondria	less abundant than in ventricular cell	most abundant	less abundant than in ventricular cell
Glycogen	present between myofibrils with mitochondria		characteristic large pools both intermyofibrillar and subsarcolemmal
Granules	"atrial granules": function and composition unknown	"residual bodies": high in catecholamine content	
Transverse Tubular System	absent	abundant	absent
Sarcoplasmic reticulum	well developed and abundant in all cell types		
INTERCELLULAR LINKAGES Intercalated discs	Short, horizontally oriented to long axis of cell. Less frequent, short perpendicularly oriented discs.	Characteristic stepwise configuration with nonspecialized portions horizontal to long axis of myofiber and specialized areas perpendicular to long axis of myofiber: principally end-to-end links between cells	Oblique and zigzag course. Highest proportion of specialized linkage with greatest surface are of all 3 cell types.
Side-to-side	principal location of cell-to-cell connections	Brief, infrequent	abundant

Specific References

1. James, T. N., Sherf, L., Fine, G., and Morales, A. R.: Comparative Ultrastructure of the Sinus Node in Man and Dog. *Circ.*, 34:139, 1966.
2. James, T. N.: Anatomy of the AV Node of the Dog. *Anat. Rec.*, 148:15, 1964.
3. Miller, J. P., Wallace, A. G., and Feezor, M. D.: A Quantitative Comparison of the Relation Between the Shape of the Action Potential and the Pattern of Stimulation in Canine Ventricular Muscle and Purkinje Fibers. *J. Mol. Cell. Cardiol.*, 2:3, 1971.
4. Jamieson, J. D. and Palade, G. G.: Specific Granules in Atrial Muscle Cells. *J. Cell. Biol.*, 23:151, 1964.
5. Berger, J. M. and Bencosme, S. A.: Fine Structural Cytochemistry of Granules in Atrial Cardiocytes. *J. Mol. Cell. Cardiol.*, 3:111, 1971.
6. Palade, G. E.: Secretory Granules in Atrial Myocardium. *Anat. Rec.*, 139:262, 1961.
7. Weidmann, S.: Electrical Constants of Trabecular Muscle from Mammalian Heart. *J. Physiol.*, 210:1041, 1970.
8. Weidmann, S.: The Electrical Constants of Purkinje Fibers. *J. Physiol.*, 118:348, 1952.
9. Weidmann, S.: The Diffusion of Radiopotassium across Intercalated Discs of Mammalian Cardiac Muscle. *J. Physiol. (London)*, 187:323, 1966.
10. Berger, J. M. and Rona, G.: Fine Structure of Extranodal Transitional Cardiocytes in Rat Left Atrium. *J. Mol. Cell. Cardiol.*, 2:181, 1971.

Index

and excitation-contraction coupling 81
in pathologic states, 89
differences between skeletal and cardiac, 80, 82
difference between mitochondrial and sarcoplasmic reticulum uptake, 91

Sodium
competition with calcium, 13
flux across membrane, 20
Specific granule, 133
Supernormal period, 21

Thick filaments, 6, 12, 37
bare area, 46
Thin filaments, 6, 12, 35
active sites, 54
Tight junction, 32
Transcription, 93
Transitional cell, 1
Translation, 93
Transmembrane potential, 17

Transverse tubular system, 21
and the extracellular space, 21
as a sarcolemmal derivative, 6
role in excitation-contraction coupling, 21
and the afterpotential, 21
Triad, 6
Tropomyosin, 36
A, 36
B, 36
Troponin, 36, 37

Uncoupled cell, 12
Unit membrane theory, 13
see also 'membrane'

Ventricular Cell
action potential, 12, 17
morphology, 155
Voltage clamping, 16

Z-Band, 6, 35, 36
Z substance in sarcomerogenesis, 103-104
polarity, 103

THE LIBRARY
UNIVERSITY OF CALIFORNIA
San Francisco
THIS BOOK IS DUE ON THE LAST DATE STAMPED BELOW

Books not returned on time are subject to fines according to the Library
Lending Code. A renewal may be made on certain materials. For details
consult Lending Code.